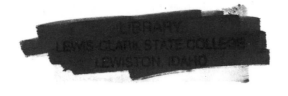

Practical Guide to Exercise Physiology

Practical Guide to Exercise Physiology

Bob Murray, PhD

Sports Science Insights, LLC

W. Larry Kenney, PhD

Pennsylvania State University, University Park

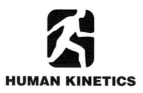

HUMAN KINETICS

Library of Congress Cataloging-in-Publication Data

Murray, Robert, 1949- , author.
 Practical guide to exercise physiology / Bob Murray, W. Larry Kenney.
    p. ; cm.
 Includes index.
 I. Kenney, W. Larry, author. II. Title.
 [DNLM: 1. Exercise--physiology. 2. Exercise Movement Techniques. 3. Physical Exertion. QT 256]
 RA781
 613.7'1--dc23

                              2015020548

 ISBN: 978-1-4504-6180-1 (print)

The web addresses cited in this text were current as of September 2, 2015, unless otherwise noted.

Acquisitions Editor: Amy N. Tocco; **Developmental Editor:** Katherine Maurer; **Managing Editor:** B. Rego; **Copyeditor:** Jan Feeney; **Indexer:** Laurel Plotzke; **Permissions Manager:** Dalene Reeder; **Graphic Designer:** Nancy Rasmus; **Cover Designer:** Keith Blomberg; **Photograph (cover):** © Human Kinetics; photo by Jason Allen and anatomical art by Jennifer Gibas; **Photographs (interior):** © Human Kinetics, unless otherwise noted; **Photo Asset Manager:** Laura Fitch; **Visual Production Assistant:** Joyce Brumfield; **Photo Production Manager:** Jason Allen; **Art Manager:** Kelly Hendren; **Associate Art Manager:** Alan L. Wilborn; **Art Style Development:** Joanne Brummett and Jennifer Gibas; **Illustrations:** © Human Kinetics unless otherwise noted; **Printer:** Versa Press

Printed in the United States of America   10 9 8 7 6 5 4 3 2 1

The paper in this book is certified under a sustainable forestry program.

Human Kinetics
Website: www.HumanKinetics.com

United States: Human Kinetics
P.O. Box 5076
Champaign, IL 61825-5076
800-747-4457
e-mail: info@hkusa.com

Canada: Human Kinetics
475 Devonshire Road Unit 100
Windsor, ON N8Y 2L5
800-465-7301 (in Canada only)
e-mail: info@hkcanada.com

Europe: Human Kinetics
107 Bradford Road
Stanningley
Leeds LS28 6AT, United Kingdom
+44 (0) 113 255 5665
e-mail: hk@hkeurope.com

Australia: Human Kinetics
57A Price Avenue
Lower Mitcham, South Australia 5062
08 8372 0999
e-mail: info@hkaustralia.com

New Zealand: Human Kinetics
P.O. Box 80
Mitcham Shopping Centre, South Australia 5062
0800 222 062
e-mail: info@hknewzealand.com

E6026

|CONTENTS

Preface vii
Acknowledgments ix
Photo Credits xi

PART I   Warming Up: Physiology 101

ONE   Muscles Move Us   3
How Do Muscles Work? 4
How Do Muscles Adapt to Training? 12
How Do Muscle Cells Get Bigger and Stronger? 20

TWO   Food Really Is Fuel   23
From Food to Energy 24
How Do Nutrients Fuel Muscle? 27
What About Vitamins and Minerals? 39
Water Is a Nutrient, Too 41

THREE   Muscles Need Oxygen   45
How Does Oxygen Get to Muscles? 46
How Does Oxygen Use Relate to Fitness and Energy Expenditure? 49
How Does Training Help the Body Use More Oxygen? 54
Oxygen Delivery and Performance Enhancement 58

FOUR   Fatigue: What Is It Good For?   61
What Causes Fatigue? 62
What's the Difference Between Fatigue and Overtraining? 72
What Role Does Fatigue Play in Adaptations to Training? 75

PART II   The Science of Training Program Design

FIVE   Principles of Designing Training Programs   79
What Are the Basics of Program Design? 80
What Makes an Effective Training Program? 85
Training Terms 91

SIX   **Training to Improve Muscle Mass and Strength**   **93**

How Do Strength and Mass Increase? 94
What's the Best Way to Gain Strength and Mass? 97
What's the Role of Nutrition? 105

SEVEN   **Training for Weight Loss**   **107**

Weight Loss Is All About Energy Balance 108
Why Do Some People Have Difficulty Losing Weight? 118
What's the Best Way to Lose Fat but Protect Muscle Mass? 120

EIGHT   **Training for Speed and Power**   **125**

What Are Speed and Power? 126
What Adaptations Are Needed to Improve Speed and Power? 128
What Kinds of Training Improve Speed and Power? 130
What Does a Speed and Power Training Session Look Like? 136

NINE   **Training for Aerobic Endurance**   **139**

What Are the Main Adaptations to Aerobic Training? 140
What's the Best Way to Improve Aerobic Endurance? 148
Should Endurance Athletes Engage in Strength Training? 151
Why Is Endurance Capacity Important for Sprinters and
  Team-Sport Athletes? 152

PART III Special Considerations

TEN   **Heat, Cold, and Altitude**   **155**

Exercise in the Heat Impairs Performance 156
Cold Stress Chills Performance 163
Exercise at Altitude 165

ELEVEN   **Training Children, Older Adults, and Pregnant Women**   **171**

Do Children Respond Differently Than Adults
  to Exercise Training? 172
Can Children Improve Strength With Training? 175
Can Older Adults Adapt to Training? 179
Should Women Exercise During Pregnancy? 183

Index of Common Questions From Clients 185
Index 189
About the Authors 195

You are likely a strong believer in the benefits of regular exercise and are interested in learning more about how the body responds to exercise and training. In your quest for knowledge, you should be aware that there are many excellent exercise physiology textbooks to choose from. In fact, Dr. Kenney is the coauthor of one of the best-selling exercise physiology textbooks for undergraduate students, *Physiology of Sport and Exercise, Sixth Edition* (Kenney, Wilmore, & Costill, Human Kinetics 2012).

We decided to write a different kind of exercise physiology textbook, one that is long on illustrations and short on text, because we understand that busy sport fitness professionals need quick and easy access to accurate and up-to-date scientific information. This text is intended for a variety of people, from those new to the field who want to learn the fundamentals of exercise physiology to professionals who have taken exercise physiology classes in the past and acquired certifications but need to quickly refresh their memories about the scientific underpinnings of exercise and sport.

This book provides an easy, straightforward way for you to review the principles of exercise physiology or learn something new that you can put to immediate use in your own training. It will also help you refine or design training programs or educate others about the ability of the human body to respond and adapt to regular physical activity. Whether the goal of exercise is to lose weight or gain strength, speed, or stamina, understanding how the body responds physiologically to the stress of exercise should be basic knowledge for all sport fitness professionals.

Organization of the Book

Practical Guide to Exercise Physiology is divided into three parts. Part I covers how the muscles, heart, lung, and nervous system respond to exercise and training, how food and drink are converted to fuel, how oxygen enables the breakdown of food into fuel, and how fatigue limits the capacity for exercise.

Part II focuses on the design of training programs by reviewing the principles that should be the basis of every training program and then highlighting specific design features for programs tailored to improve mass and strength, speed weight loss, enhance speed and power, and maximize aerobic endurance.

Part III is devoted to special considerations such as training clients and athletes to withstand the rigors of heat, cold, altitude, and air pollution. Also covered is the design of training programs for children, older adults, and pregnant women.

Special Features

In addition to the numerous photos and detailed illustrations, *Practical Guide to Exercise Physiology* contains special features to make the science come alive in practical form:

- Scientific terms and concepts are defined and explained using everyday language.
- Numerous examples help you apply physiology as you help clients meet their goals.
- Art and photos integrated with the content provide an engaging, highly visual reading experience.
- Sidebars highlight important topics and common questions in exercise physiology.
- Fun facts add interest throughout the text.
- The index of common questions from clients is a quick reference to help you educate clients.

If you have little background in exercise science, *Practical Guide to Exercise Physiology* gets you started on your sport science journey. And if you have taken classes in exercise physiology, this text will quickly refresh your memory about the fundamental concepts and practical applications of the science related to human physiology, metabolism, and nutrition. We hope the information in this book makes that science come alive for you and your clients.

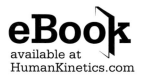

eBook
available at
HumanKinetics.com

We would like to express our appreciation to the staff at Human Kinetics for their foresight in identifying the opportunity for this book, their persistence in nudging us to write it, and their unending patience in getting us to finish it. Special thanks to Amy Tocco and Kate Maurer for shepherding us through the process from start to finish. Additional thanks to Joanne Brummett for her artistic guidance in creating illustrations that bring the science to life in simple, understandable ways.

And last, but certainly not least, unending thanks to our families, who endured our absences during the many hours required to finish this project. The fact that no one complained much about the amount of time we spent on this book is testimony to their patience, love, and support. Or perhaps they were just happy that we were busy enough to leave them alone. Either way, we very much appreciate the opportunity they helped make possible.

Bob Murray
W. Larry Kenney

Chapter 1

Chapter opening photo © MR.BIG-PHOTOGRAPHY/iStock
Man rock climbing, p. 5, © Doug Olson/Fotolia
Muscle micrograph in figure 1.5, p.10, reprinted from W.L. Kenney, J.H. Willmore, and D.L. Costill, 2015, *Physiology of sport and exercise*, 6th ed. (Champaign, IL: Human Kinetics), 39. By permission of D.L. Costill.
Suspension training, p. 13, © Christopher Futcher/iStock
Stationary cycling, p. 14, © ferrantraite/iStock
Woman on elliptical machine, p. 15 © Andres Rodriguez/Fotolia
Barbell training, p. 17, © Bananastock

Chapter 2

Chapter opening photo © standret/iStock
Woman with dumbbells, p. 25, © Bananastock
Bread, p. 26, © diegofrias/iStock
Bacon, p. 26, © Nirad/iStock
Steak, p. 26, © Alex Kladoff/iStock
Drinking water, p. 42, © 2001 Brand X Pictures
Worker in the heat, p. 43, © Associated Press

Chapter 3

Chapter opening photo © technotr/iStock
Sedentary woman, p. 51, © davide cerati/Age fotostock
Cross-country skier, p. 51, © Gepa Pictures/Imago/Icon Sportswire
Football player, p. 58, © Chris Williams/Icon Sportswire

Chapter 4

Chapter opening photo © Jacob Ammentorp Lund/iStock
Sprinters, p. 63, © Julien Crosnier/KMSP/DPPI/Icon Sportswire
Fatigued athlete with water, p. 66, © BartekSzewczyk/iStock
Weary athlete with barbell, p. 74, © Martin Dimitrov/iStock

Chapter 5

Chapter opening photo © Predrag Vuckovic/iStock
Man on treadmill, p. 87, © Bananastock

Chapter 6

Kayaker, p. 95, © Getty Images
Dumbbell tricep exercise, p. 97, © Anton/Fotolia
Electrical muscle training device, p. 104, © Kyodo/AP images
Sandwich, p. 105, © miflippo/iStock
Cottage cheese, p. 105, © Og-vision/iStock

Chapter 7

Chapter opening photo CO 07 © Clubfoot/iStock
Bear, p. 111, © Dieter Meyrl/iStock

Chapter 8

Chapter opening photo © Chris Cheadle/Age fotostock
Football players, p. 127, © Jeff Mills/Icon Sportswire
Volleyball player, p. 127, © John S. Peterson/Icon Sportswire
Sprinter, p. 127, © technotr/iStock
Javelin throw, p. 128, MOCK © Becky Miller/Gopher Track Shots
Recreational softball, p. 130, © George Shelley/Age fotostock
Stair running, p. 132, © Matt Brown/iStock
Stationary cycling, p. 135, © Amana Productions, Inc. /Age fotostock

Chapter 9

Chapter opening photo © Serge Simo/Fotolia.com
Woman jumping hurdle, p. 143, © Microgen/iStock
Wilson Kipsang Kiprotich, p. 144, © Zuma Press/Icon Sportswire
Man biking in mountains, p. 145, © Maxim Petrichuk/Fotolia
Jump training, p. 148, © Xavier Arnau/iStock
Hill running, p. 150, © Michael Svoboda/iStock

Chapter 10

Chapter opening photo © Einstein
Infrared images, p. 156, Department of Health and Human Performance, Auburn
  University, Alabama. Courtesy of John Eric Smith, Joe Molloy, and David D.
  Pascoe. By permission of David Pascoe.
Photo in figure 10.3 © Ed Wolfstein/Icon Sportswire
Fatigued cyclist, p. 161, © Vincent Curutchet/DPPI/Icon Sportswire
Photo in figure 10.4 © Andrea Strauss/Age fotostock
Cyclists at altitude, p. 168, © Gorfer/iStock

Chapter 11

Chapter opening photo © Kevin Dodge/Age footstock
Arm scans in figure 11.6 from W.L. Kenney, J.H. Wilmore, and D.L. Costill,
  2015. *Physiology of sport and exercise*, 6th ed. (Champaign, IL: Human Kinetics).
Senior woman with dumbbell, p. 182, © Alfred Wekelo/Fotolia
Pregnant women, p. 183, © kate_sept2004/iStock

PART I

Warming Up: Physiology 101

CHAPTER ONE

Muscles Move Us

When you train muscles, you also train the systems that support them.

Exercise physiology is the study of how the body responds to exercise and physical training, so what better place to start this book than with skeletal muscle, the engines that move the body? During exercise, the muscles take center stage. While you're also aware that heart rate has increased and breathing becomes heavier, it's natural that you're most tuned in to your muscles. After all, it's the muscles you're trying to change with exercise training. You might want your muscles to be stronger, or bigger, or more defined, or more flexible, or more agile, or faster, or you might want them to have more endurance. With proper training, any of those improvements are possible. But muscles cannot function in isolation, and as you train the muscles, you're also training the nervous system, heart, lungs, blood vessels, liver, kidneys, and many other organs and tissues. Planning an effective training program requires keeping in mind that big picture—a picture that involves more than just muscles.

But because muscle is the foundation for movement, a review of muscle physiology 101 is a great place to start.

How Do Muscles Work?

Take a quick look at figure 1.1. Similar figures appear in many textbooks because certain basic parts to skeletal muscle are important to recognize. When talking about muscle, you most likely think of skeletal muscles because those are the muscles that are involved in exercise and you can feel them working and tiring and aching. But cardiac muscle in the heart and smooth muscle in blood vessels and the gastrointestinal tract are also very much involved in supporting the body's ability to exercise. Cardiac muscle and smooth muscle have different structures and functions. The focus here is on skeletal muscle, the muscles that move the body.

Skeletal muscles are roughly 75% water. In other words, if you gain 10 pounds of muscle tissue, you actually gain 7.5 pounds of water and 2.5 pounds of contractile proteins and other cellular components.

▌FIGURE 1.1 The structure of muscle.

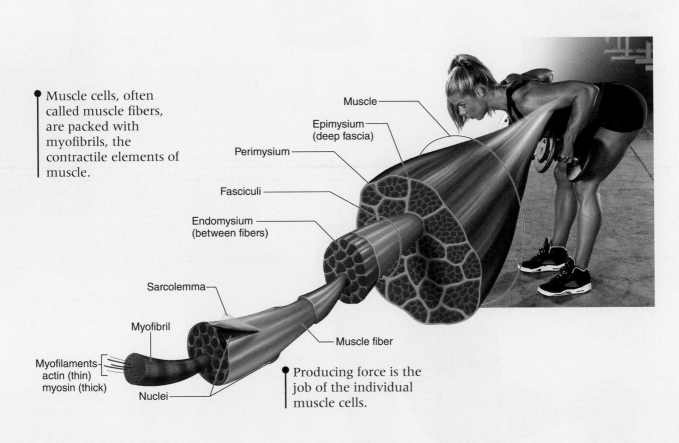

Muscle cells, often called muscle fibers, are packed with myofibrils, the contractile elements of muscle.

Muscle

Epimysium (deep fascia)

Perimysium

Fasciculi

Endomysium (between fibers)

Sarcolemma

Myofibril

Myofilaments
actin (thin)
myosin (thick)

Nuclei

Muscle fiber

Producing force is the job of the individual muscle cells.

Even though skeletal muscles come in many shapes and sizes, they all share a common internal structure. Skeletal muscles are simply bundles of individual muscle cells (called fasciculi) arranged in groups controlled by individual nerves (alpha motor neuron; see figure 1.2) so that all the cells in the group contract in unison. Each muscle cell is packed with contractile proteins (the myofibrils actin and myosin), enzymes (to help speed up reactions), nuclei (for protein production), mitochondria (for energy production), glycogen (the storage form of glucose used by the cell for energy), and sarcoplasmic reticulum (to aid contraction and relaxation; see figure 1.4). The structure of each cell is supported on the inside by a framework of proteins and on the outside by various types of connective tissues that support individual cells, bundles of cells, and the entire muscle. The terms *endomysium*, *perimysium*, and *epimysium* refer to these connective tissues.

The basic job of muscle is to move bones around their joints. This requires that muscles contract with enough force to get that job done, whether that entails lifting a heavy weight once, sprinting a short distance, or cycling a long distance.

Motor units in the muscles controlling eye movements may contain as few as 10 muscle cells.

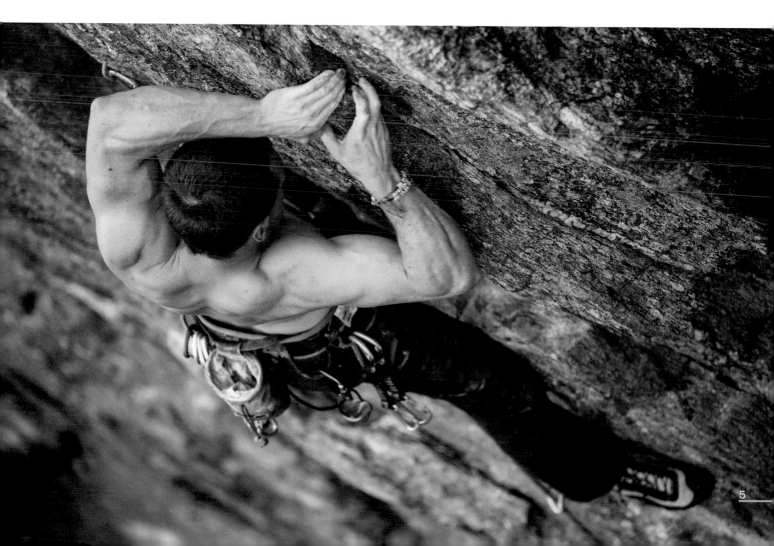

The Electrical Connection

Skeletal muscle fibers don't contract on their own but usually require input from the brain (though some reflex movements involve spinal nerves and muscles). Figure 1.2 is a simple illustration of one nerve (a motor neuron) connected to three muscle cells. The motor neuron and its attached muscle cells are referred to as a motor unit. A single motor neuron may be connected to (innervate) dozens, or hundreds, or even thousands of individual muscle cells, depending on the size and function of the muscle. When the motor neuron fires, all of the muscle cells in that motor unit contract maximally. For movements that require little strength, such as picking up a fork, only a few motor units are activated. For movements that require maximal strength, a maximal number of available motor units are activated. When an untrained person begins strength training, most of the initial improvement in muscle strength over the first couple months is due to increased recruitment of motor units by the central nervous system, a good example of how muscles operate in cooperation with other organ systems.

It's important to understand how nerves cause muscles to contract because if that process is disrupted, strength is impaired, as detailed in chapter 4. Figure 1.3 is a simple overview of the various steps required for muscle to contract, which will give you a basic understanding (or review) of how skeletal muscle cells contract.

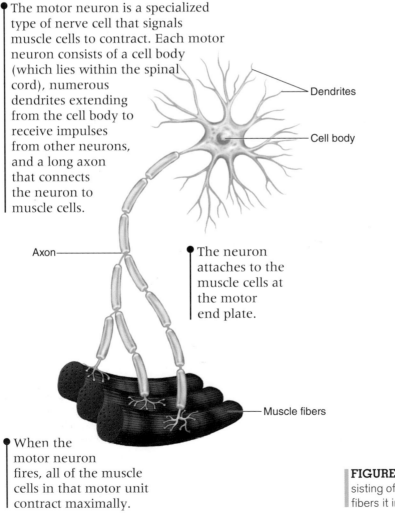

● The motor neuron is a specialized type of nerve cell that signals muscle cells to contract. Each motor neuron consists of a cell body (which lies within the spinal cord), numerous dendrites extending from the cell body to receive impulses from other neurons, and a long axon that connects the neuron to muscle cells.

Dendrites

Cell body

Axon

● The neuron attaches to the muscle cells at the motor end plate.

Muscle fibers

● When the motor neuron fires, all of the muscle cells in that motor unit contract maximally.

FIGURE 1.2 A motor unit, consisting of a motor neuron and the fibers it innervates.

∎ FIGURE 1.3 The series of events that cause muscle cells to contract.

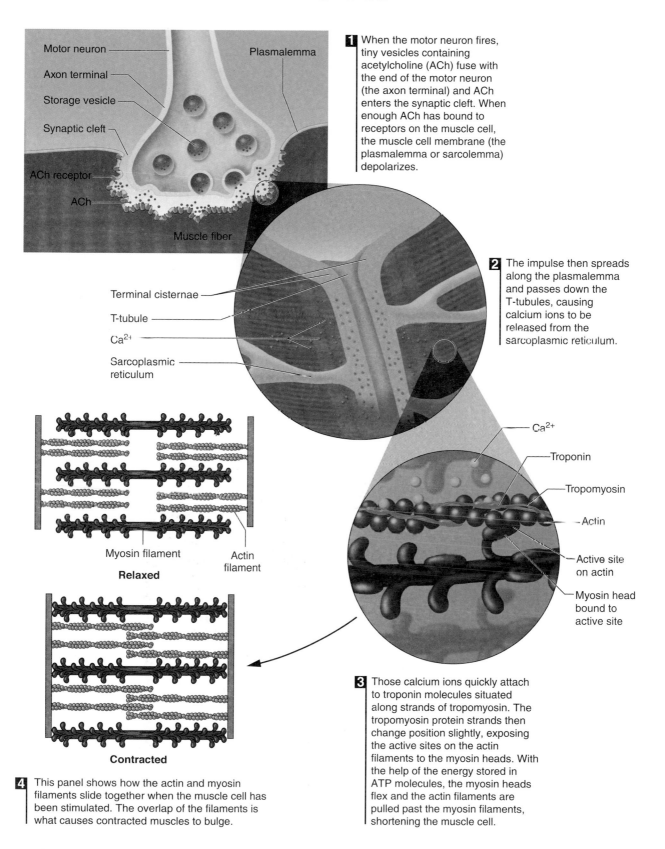

Motor neuron

Axon terminal

Storage vesicle

Synaptic cleft

ACh receptor

ACh

Plasmalemma

Muscle fiber

1 When the motor neuron fires, tiny vesicles containing acetylcholine (ACh) fuse with the end of the motor neuron (the axon terminal) and ACh enters the synaptic cleft. When enough ACh has bound to receptors on the muscle cell, the muscle cell membrane (the plasmalemma or sarcolemma) depolarizes.

Terminal cisternae

T-tubule

Ca^{2+}

Sarcoplasmic reticulum

2 The impulse then spreads along the plasmalemma and passes down the T-tubules, causing calcium ions to be released from the sarcoplasmic reticulum.

Ca^{2+}

Troponin

Tropomyosin

Actin

Active site on actin

Myosin head bound to active site

Myosin filament

Actin filament

Relaxed

Contracted

3 Those calcium ions quickly attach to troponin molecules situated along strands of tropomyosin. The tropomyosin protein strands then change position slightly, exposing the active sites on the actin filaments to the myosin heads. With the help of the energy stored in ATP molecules, the myosin heads flex and the actin filaments are pulled past the myosin filaments, shortening the muscle cell.

4 This panel shows how the actin and myosin filaments slide together when the muscle cell has been stimulated. The overlap of the filaments is what causes contracted muscles to bulge.

Here is the short version of how a muscle contracts:

First, an impulse travels from the brain to the spine and from the spine down motor neurons to the muscle cells within those motor units. At the junction between the motor neurons and each muscle cell (called the neuromuscular junction), a neurotransmitter called acetylcholine is released into the space between the nerve and the muscle (that space is called the synapse or the synaptic cleft). The impulse is thereby transmitted from the motor neuron to all the muscle cells it innervates, causing those cells to contract in unison. Before the cells contract, the impulse has to first travel across the entire muscle cell membrane (the sarcolemma or plasmalemma), dipping instantaneously into the interior of each cell through T-tubules (transverse tubules). Each impulse causes calcium ions (molecules) to be released from the sarcoplasmic reticulum; this release of calcium ions causes muscle to contract (see figure 1.3 for more detail.) When the nerve impulse stops, the calcium ions are instantly taken back into the sarcoplasmic reticulum and the muscle cells relax.

Figure 1.4 makes it clear how the plasmalemma (sarcolemma) is connected to the T-tubules and how the sarcoplas-

Some alpha motor neurons can be more than 3 feet (about one meter) long.

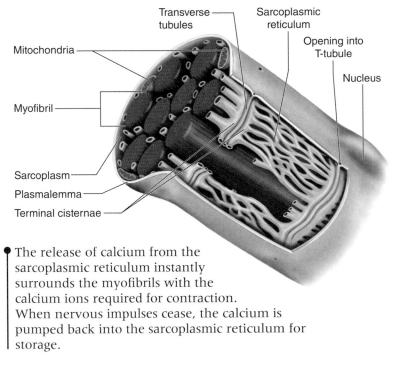

- Mitochondria
- Myofibril
- Sarcoplasm
- Plasmalemma
- Terminal cisternae
- Transverse tubules
- Sarcoplasmic reticulum
- Opening into T-tubule
- Nucleus

● The release of calcium from the sarcoplasmic reticulum instantly surrounds the myofibrils with the calcium ions required for contraction. When nervous impulses cease, the calcium is pumped back into the sarcoplasmic reticulum for storage.

FIGURE 1.4 A muscle cell is a very crowded space. Everything about the cell supports muscle contractions, from single, all-out, maximal-strength contractions to the repeated contractions needed for sustaining endurance activities.

mic reticulum (SR) surrounds the myofibrils within a single muscle cell. Jammed into the already-packed space inside muscle cells are a variety of enzymes needed for energy (ATP) production, glycogen molecules (the storage form of glucose), fat molecules, and other molecules and structures.

One of those other molecules is the protein titin. In recent years, scientists have learned that titin not only aids in maintaining the overall structure of the muscle fiber, keeping the sliding filaments (actin and myosin) in line, but it is also important in muscle strength, particularly as muscle lengthens (eccentric contractions). It seems that calcium ions cause titin to stiffen, helping to explain why muscles are so much stronger during eccentric (lengthening) contractions than during concentric (shortening) contractions. It may be that muscle cells actually contain three contractile proteins: actin, myosin, and titin.

Titin is the largest known protein, consisting of 34,350 amino acids. As a result, the formal chemical name for titin contains 189,819 letters and takes more than 3 hours to pronounce, making it the longest word in the English language.

Different Cell Types for Different Jobs

Not surprisingly, there are different types of muscle cells, a characteristic that enables humans to perform explosive movements of short duration as well as complete amazing feats of endurance exercise. The muscle fiber (cell) types are simply referred to as type I (slow twitch) and type II (fast twitch). Type I fibers are better suited for endurance exercise and type II fibers are better suited for sprints or other brief, powerful movements. Figure 1.5 shows a cross-section of muscle stained to show the different fiber types. Motor units contain only one fiber type. The motor neurons that innervate type I motor units are smaller in diameter than the neurons that supply type II motor units. In addition to that difference, type I motor units contain fewer fibers than type II motor units. As a result, type II motor units develop more force when they are activated.

Arms and legs contain a similar proportion of type I and type II muscle cells, although those proportions vary from person to person.

Type II fibers produce and use energy (ATP) faster, have a more developed sarcoplasmic reticulum (which means faster calcium cycling), and are larger than type I fibers.

Type I fibers have more mitocohondria, allowing for more sustained energy production in endurance activities.

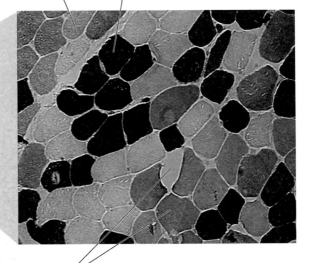

Type II muscle cells can be classified further as type IIa and type IIx, although all have similar fast-twitch characteristics.

FIGURE 1.5 Muscle cells are called on to accomplish all sorts of tasks, so it should be no surprise that cells are specialized for distinct functions.

Micrograph reprinted from W.L. Kenney, J.H. Willmore, and D.L. Costill, 2015, *Physiology of sport and exercise*, 6th ed. (Champaign, IL: Human Kinetics), 39. By permission of D.L. Costill.

Most muscles are roughly 50% fast-twitch and 50% slow-twitch, but these proportions can vary widely, as shown in table 1.1. Some elite distance runners have leg muscles in which over 90% of the muscle cells are slow-twitch (type I) fibers, while some elite sprinters have the opposite mix. Although the ratio of fiber types is determined by genetics, proper training can improve the function of any muscle cell—the very basis for greater fitness and performance.

TABLE 1.1 **Percentages and Cross-Sectional Areas of Type I and Type II Fibers in Selected Muscles of Male and Female Athletes**

Athlete	Sex	Muscle	% type I	% type II
Sprint runners	M	Gastrocnemius	24	76
	F	Gastrocnemius	27	73
Distance runners	M	Gastrocnemius	79	21
	F	Gastrocnemius	69	31
Cyclists	M	Vastus lateralis	57	43
	F	Vastus lateralis	51	49
Swimmers	M	Posterior deltoid	67	33
Weightlifters	M	Gastrocnemius	44	56
	M	Deltoid	53	47
Triathletes	M	Posterior deltoid	60	40
	M	Vastus lateralis	63	37
	M	Gastrocnemius	59	41
Canoeists	M	Posterior deltoid	71	29
Shot-putters	M	Gastrocnemius	38	62
Nonathletes	M	Vastus lateralis	47	53
	F	Gastrocnemius	52	48

Adapted, by permission, from W.L. Kenney, J.H. Wilmore, and D.L. Costill, 2015, *Physiology of sport and exercise*, 6th ed. (Champaign, IL: Human Kinetics), 45.

What Happens When Muscles Stretch?

Why do muscles feel tight whenever they are stretched? For example, when you try to touch your toes while the knees are locked, the hamstring muscles stretch and you feel that tension. But what causes the tension? For many decades, the prevailing theory was that the passive tension produced when a muscle is stretched was due to an increased tension in the connective tissues surrounding the muscles. It turns out those connective tissues may not be responsible for the forces produced when a muscle is stretched. Eccentric muscle contractions stretch muscle cells, reducing the opportunity for actin and myosin to interact. Yet eccentric contractions are very powerful. Recent research has shown that the structural protein titin may play an important role in force production during eccentric contractions. Titin is an enormous protein that acts like a spring inside each skeletal muscle cell. Stretch the cell and the titin molecules are also stretched. Just as a rubber band increases its tension when stretched, so does titin, adding to the force produced by actin and myosin. In that regard, titin may be considered the third contractile protein in muscle cells.

How Do Muscles Adapt to Training?

In the simplest terms, when muscles are stressed by exercise, they gradually increase their capacity to handle that stress. For instance, muscles adapt to strength training by increasing the number of motor units that are recruited during weightlifting and by producing more myofibrillar protein (actin, myosin, and other proteins involved in muscle contraction). Those changes result in increased strength and often increased muscle size. With endurance training, muscles adapt by increasing the number and size of energy-producing mitochondria as well as the enzymes used to break down glycogen, glucose, and fatty acids for energy.

All of these adaptations occur because regular training results in changes in the many nuclei contained in each muscle cell. The DNA in the nucleus of every muscle cell contains genes that are the blueprints for every protein within a muscle cell, such as contractile proteins, structural proteins, regulatory proteins, mitochondrial proteins, and enzymes. With training, changes in gene expression in the cell lead to increased levels of functional proteins.

As depicted in figure 1.6, the adaptations that eventually result from the stimulus of exercise training require a variety of facilitators to maximize the response. For example, the response to training will be less than optimal if the client or athlete is chronically dehydrated, eats poorly, and doesn't get enough rest. Optimal response to training is made possible by the nervous, immune, and hormonal (endocrine) systems, all of which are disrupted by poor hydration, nutrition, and rest. In other words, for optimal responses to occur, a great training program has to be complemented by proper hydration, nutrition, and rest.

Genetics also plays a large role in the adaptations that result from training. Everyone adapts uniquely to exercise training because everyone has a unique genetic makeup. Genes determine the speed and magnitude of the

FIGURE 1.6 Muscle cells adapt to the stress of training in ways that improve the muscle's capacity for exercise.

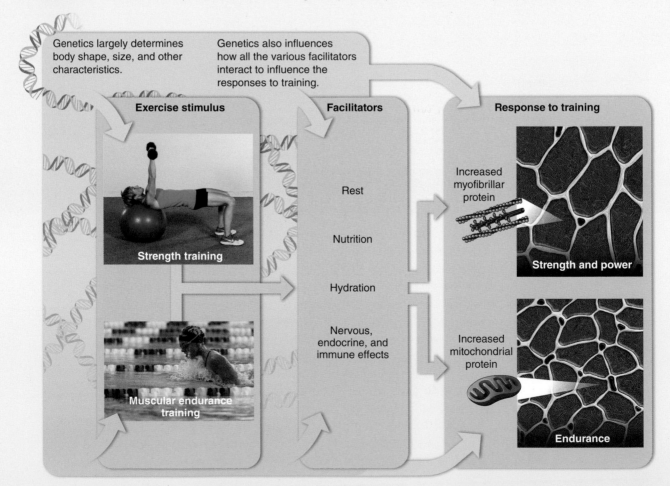

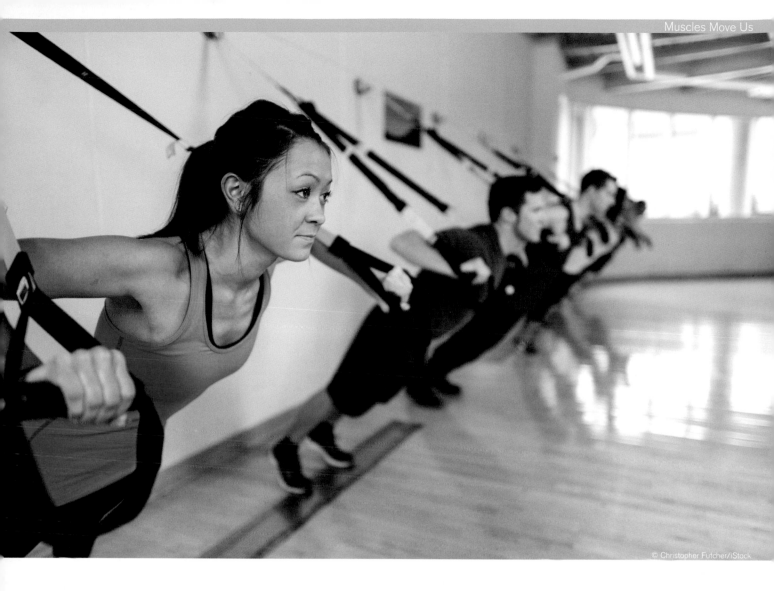

response to training. Even if every athlete or client began a training program with exactly the same strength and fitness characteristics, some would adapt to the training faster than others, making greater gains in strength, speed, and endurance. In other words, some people are high responders and some are low responders. Sex also plays a role in the capacity for adaptations to training. For example, men's muscles typically experience more hypertrophy as a result of strength training because of the greater testosterone levels in men. We'll learn more about these differences later in this book.

Genetics plays a large role in adaptation because genetic makeup determines the upper limits of strength, speed, and endurance. For example, research has shown that 25% to 50% of maximal oxygen uptake ($\dot{V}O_{2max}$) is determined by genetics. The painful truth is that no matter how hard some people train, the highest $\dot{V}O_{2max}$ they may be able to attain might be lower than that of an untrained individual who has the genetic predisposition for a high $\dot{V}O_{2max}$. The same is true for strength, speed, agility, flexibility, and other athletic characteristics.

If genes determine only part of the ability to adapt to training, what determines the other part? That's where work ethic, dedication, rest, nutrition, and hydration enter the picture. The adaptations that result from exercise training require months of consistent hard work. That regular overload on the muscle, combined with adequate rest, proper hydration, and ample nutrition create and support the intracellular environment that optimizes the production of all the functional proteins that are needed for increased strength, speed, and stamina.

Contracting muscles also operate as a muscle pump that assists the return of blood to the heart through the veins.

Adaptations to Aerobic, Anaerobic, and Strength Training

Muscles are the engines that move the body, and like all engines, muscles have to be fueled and cooled, and waste products have to be removed. Those jobs fall to the lungs, heart, vasculature, liver, and kidneys with the help of endocrine glands (such as the pituitary, hypothalamus, thyroid, pancreas, and adrenal

Adaptations to Aerobic Training

In the Heart

Increased size of the heart (cardiac hypertrophy)

Increased thickness of the heart's left ventricle

Reduced resting heart rate

Faster recovery of heart rate after exercise bouts

Increased stroke volume (the volume of blood per heart beat)

Increased maximal cardiac output (the volume of blood pumped by the heart each minute)

In the Muscles

Increased maximal oxygen uptake ($\dot{V}O_{2max}$)

Increased endurance capacity

Increased oxygen extraction from the blood by active muscles

Increased enzymes involved in energy (ATP) production from carbohydrate and fat

Increased muscle and liver glycogen content

Increased cross-sectional area of type I muscle cells

Increased muscle myoglobin content

Increased number and size of muscle cell mitochondria

Increased lactate threshold

Increased maximal lactate production

Increased reliance on fatty acids for fuel at submaximal intensities

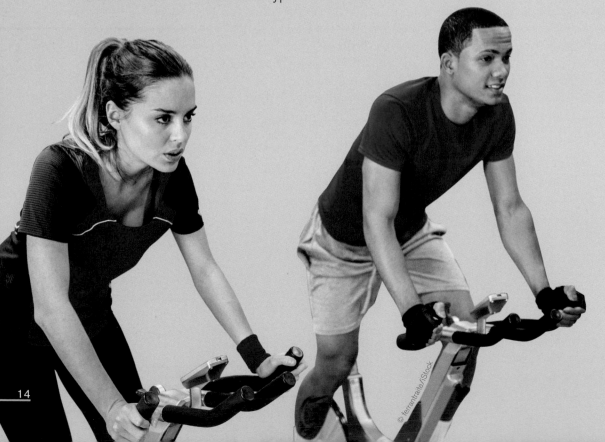

©ferrantraite/iStock

glands). As muscles adapt to training, so do the tissues and organs that support muscle function.

Following is a list of many of the adaptations that result from aerobic (endurance) training, all of which help support the continued contraction of skeletal muscle during endurance exercise. This long list of adaptations is evidence that exercise is powerful stuff when it comes to promoting changes that improve health and performance.

In the Circulation

Increased plasma volume (the fluid portion of the blood)

Increased number of red blood cells (RBCs)

Increased blood volume (plasma volume + RBCs)

Reduced resting blood pressure in those with high blood pressure

Increased maximal blood pressure (systolic)

Reduced blood pressure during submaximal exercise

Increased blood flow to active muscles and skin

Better redistribution of blood from inactive tissues to active muscles and skin

Increased muscle blood flow (an increase in the number of capillaries and greater activation of existing capillaries)

In the Lungs

Increased maximal ventilation of the lungs (greater tidal volume and respiratory rate)

Increased diffusion of O_2 and CO_2 in the lungs

Training for sprint and power events in sports

such as running, swimming, soccer, football, basketball, wrestling, volleyball, boxing, hockey, and rugby produces some of the same adaptations as seen with endurance training, but other adaptations occur that are better suited to meet the demands of all-out activities of fairly short duration. This list includes many of the adaptations that occur as a result of anaerobic training programs.

Anaerobic training programs can also be effective at improving aerobic capacity and performance. That's not to say that endurance athletes should switch training programs to emphasize anaerobic training, but endurance athletes can improve their speed and power without sacrificing their aerobic fitness. Another practical benefit of anaerobic training of fairly short duration (for example, a 10-minute warm-up followed by six 30-second sprints separated by 3 minutes of rest) is that improvements in both anaerobic and aerobic capacity can be had with very

Adaptations to Anaerobic Training

In the Muscles

Improved anaerobic power and capacity

Improved aerobic power and capacity

Increased muscle strength

Increased size of type II fibers

Increased size of type I fibers but less so than type II

Small increase in the percentage of type II fibers

Increased ATP-PCr enzyme activities

Increased glycolytic enzyme activities

Increased enzymes involved in aerobic ATP production (Krebs cycle)

In the Bone

Increased bone mineral density and bone strength

Increased strength of ligaments and tendons

little investment in exercise time, a real benefit for anyone who finds it difficult to set aside an hour or two for daily workouts. We revisit this topic in chapter 8. Strength training produces just the kinds of adaptations that you might expect. As mentioned earlier in this chapter, much of the initial gain in strength results from changes in the central nervous system that promote increased recruitment of motor units. Subsequent increases in strength and mass occur over weeks and months as muscles lay down more contractile proteins. Most types of training also benefit bone and ligaments, and that is especially true of activities that involve weight bearing or repeated high impact. Good examples are running, gymnastics, strength training, and power training. Cycling, swimming, and other sports in which there is little stress on bones may actually hamper bone development and strength, an additional reason that cross-training can be beneficial.

Adaptations to Strength Training

In the Muscle

More motor units recruited

Greater stimulation frequency of motor units

More synchronous recruiting of motor units

Reduced inhibition of motor units

Increased muscle cell size (hypertrophy)

Possibly a small increase in the number of muscle cells (hyperplasia)

In the Bone

Increased bone mineral density and bone strength

Increased strength of ligaments and tendons

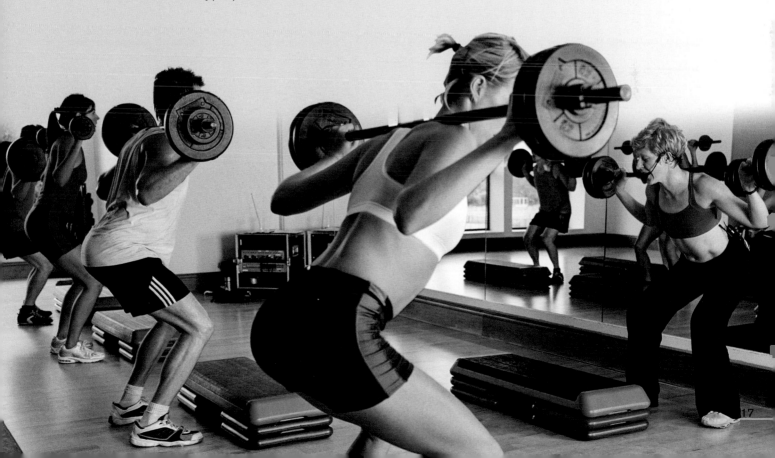

Is Damage Required for Maximizing Adaptation?

The short answer is that yes, minor damage to the muscle fibers appears to be involved in positive adaptations, but a little background information will keep things in perspective. Although the mantra "no pain, no gain" is bad advice that can result in injury or worse, might periodic muscle damage be needed for stimulating muscle to produce more contractile proteins and greater strength? Almost everyone has experienced the acute muscle soreness that accompanies vigorous exercise, especially high-intensity exercise, but those feelings of soreness and discomfort usually subside within minutes after exercise. The muscle soreness that lingers after exercise or arises a day or two later is referred to as delayed-onset muscle soreness (DOMS) and indicates damaged muscle.

DOMS is caused by eccentric muscle activity such as downhill running, lowering a heavy weight, or repeated jumps from a platform. DOMS can also occur after any activity that is new and different because virtually all movements involve some eccentric contractions. In each example, muscles resist lengthening, resulting in ruptured muscle cell membranes and disrupted alignment of contractile proteins, as shown in figure 1.7. Edema (swelling of the damaged area) and inflammation are also hallmarks of DOMS, as fluid and immune cells move from the blood into the muscle to clean up the damage and make way for new proteins.

DOMS temporarily reduces muscle strength because of the damage to contractile proteins and impairs the restoration of muscle glycogen until the damage is repaired. But might periodic DOMS actually be good for stimulating muscle hypertrophy? There are many ways in which muscles become larger, and it is possible that muscle damage can stimulate these adaptations. Research shows that muscle hypertrophy is greater with eccentric exercise training than with concentric training. Interestingly, muscle hypertrophy has been reported to be greater with rapid-velocity eccentric training, perhaps because of greater muscle damage. That finding does not suggest that eccentric training should be the only way to strength train, but this research does underscore the importance of including periodic eccentric training (and DOMS) when increases in mass and strength are desired.

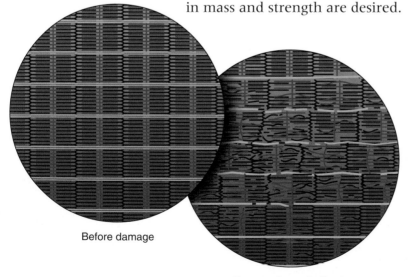

Severe damage disrupts the contractile filaments, resulting in an inflammatory response and pain.

Strength is reduced until the damage is repaired.

Before damage

Damaged muscle fibers

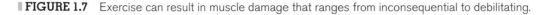

FIGURE 1.7　Exercise can result in muscle damage that ranges from inconsequential to debilitating.

What Happens When Muscles Cramp, and How Can You Avoid It?

You've had muscle cramps of one sort or another. Usually those cramps amount to little more than a temporary nuisance or, at worst, cause you to stop exercising for the day. Muscle cramps are a good example of how muscle function is integrated with CNS activity and nutrition.

Let's start with three things that scientists know about muscle cramps: (1) not all muscle cramps are the same, (2) there is no single cause for muscle cramps; and (3) for those reasons, there is no one way to prevent muscle cramping.

The most common muscle cramp is when a single muscle group contracts and remains contracted, causing immediate, localized pain. Examples are cramped calf muscles in runners or cyclists, cramped hamstrings in football players, cramped muscles in the feet of swimmers, and cramped leg muscles during sleep.

Some cramps appear to be caused by an overstimulation of nerve input to muscles. Others likely occur from dehydration or a combination of dehydration and salt loss in sweat. The cramps that swimmers have in their feet are likely caused by local fatigue resulting from keeping their toes pointed while they swim. The cramping that can occur during sleep and other nonexercise occasions may be due to nerve–muscle imbalance (more about that in a bit). Whole-body muscle cramps—sometimes called "heat cramps," and the worst of all cramping—are thought to result from dehydration and salt loss during high-intensity or prolonged exercise.

The very nature of a muscle cramp indicates that there is an imbalance in the normal interaction between the motor nerve and the muscle. Muscles contract only in response to nerve input, so a sustained cramp is evidence of sustained, abnormal input from the nerves supplying that muscle.

In 1878, doctors noticed that gold miners in Nevada were prone to whole-body muscle cramps. The same with workers on the Hoover Dam and with coal shovelers on steam ships. In all cases, the cramps were prevented when the workers increased their fluid and salt intake. Staying well hydrated, well fueled (with carbohydrate), and well salted (with electrolytes) prevents the muscle cramping associated with dehydration, fatigue, and salt loss.

Once cramps hit, there is little to do but to stop exercise and stretch (or be stretched). Severe, whole-body muscle cramps often require intravenous saline infusion and a prescription muscle relaxant. Other cramp remedies include drinking a small volume of pickle juice, taking a taste of mustard, eating bananas or oranges, and receiving injections of calcium gluconate or magnesium sulfate. Of all those remedies, only pickle juice has some scientific evidence to support its use. Researchers think that the acetic acid (vinegar) in pickle juice stimulates receptors in the mouth and throat that help reduce the nerve input to cramped muscles. Common spices such as capsaicin or ginger may also reduce the intensity and duration of cramps.

How Do Muscle Cells Get Bigger and Stronger?

All types of exercise result in immediate changes inside and outside muscle cells that serve as signals to promote the production of new functional proteins. In response to aerobic training, the various signals result in more enzymes involved in aerobic energy production, more mitochondria to enable that energy production, and more myosin filaments with slow-twitch characteristics. Strength training signals the nuclei within muscle cells (each skeletal muscle cell contains many nuclei) to produce more contractile proteins and also wakes up satellite cells.

Reasons for Bigger Muscles (Hypertrophy)

More contractile proteins (actin and myosin)

More sarcoplasm

More myofibril units

More connective tissue

More intracellular water

What Are Satellite Cells?

All skeletal muscle cells have tiny satellite cells attached to the plasmalemma (sarcolemma). The satellite cells do nothing until they are activated by strength training, muscle damage, or muscle disease. When needed, the satellite cells spring into action, grow rapidly, and fuse into the neighboring muscle cells, leaving other satellite cells behind to meet future needs (figure 1.8). The proliferation of satellite cells is responsible for most of the muscle growth that occurs early in childhood, during puberty, and as a result of training and damage.

Satellite cells increase the content of contractile proteins in muscle cells and also the number of nuclei. Muscle cells are large cells and so require many nuclei to meet the cells' constant need for new proteins. The fitter and stronger you are, the more nuclide you have in your muscle cells. And that may be a good thing as you age because those nuclei appear to stay put over time. These additional nuclei may explain why formerly fit people who resume training improve faster than inexperienced exercisers.

▌FIGURE 1.8   Satellite cells spring into action to repair damage and promote hypertrophy.

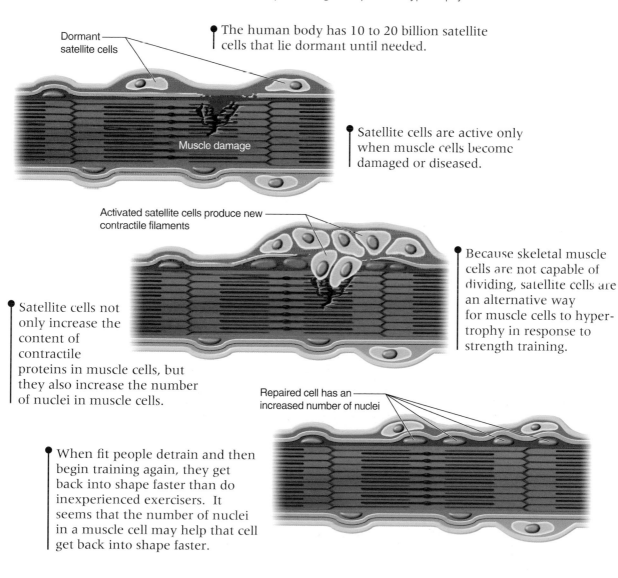

Dormant satellite cells

The human body has 10 to 20 billion satellite cells that lie dormant until needed.

Muscle damage

Satellite cells are active only when muscle cells become damaged or diseased.

Activated satellite cells produce new contractile filaments

Satellite cells not only increase the content of contractile proteins in muscle cells, but they also increase the number of nuclei in muscle cells.

Because skeletal muscle cells are not capable of dividing, satellite cells are an alternative way for muscle cells to hypertrophy in response to strength training.

Repaired cell has an increased number of nuclei

When fit people detrain and then begin training again, they get back into shape faster than do inexperienced exercisers. It seems that the number of nuclei in a muscle cell may help that cell get back into shape faster.

What Is the Role of Hormones?

Steroid and nonsteroid hormones such as testosterone, insulin, insulin-like growth factor (IGF-1), and growth hormone (GH) are among the signals that promote the production of increased functional proteins in muscle cells. Figure 1.9 shows the way that testosterone affects protein production in a muscle cell. Illegitimate use of large doses of testosterone and other anabolic steroids—including prohormones and designer steroids—results in large increases in muscle mass and strength because hormones such as testosterone continuously stimulate the production of contractile proteins.

FIGURE 1.9 Steroids and other hormones and growth factors promote the production of a variety of functional proteins inside muscle cells.

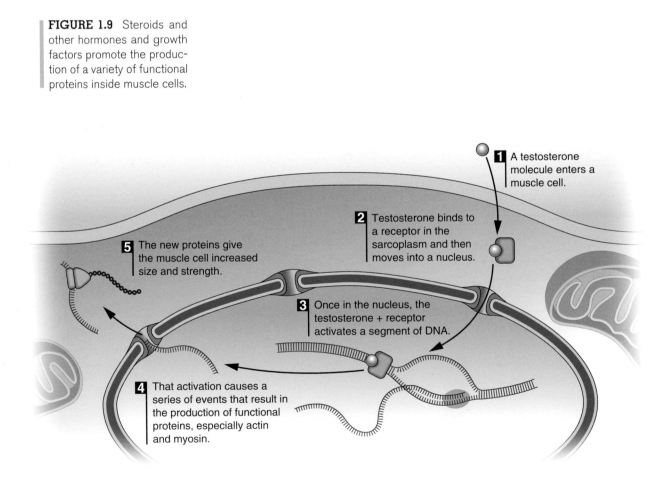

1 A testosterone molecule enters a muscle cell.

2 Testosterone binds to a receptor in the sarcoplasm and then moves into a nucleus.

3 Once in the nucleus, the testosterone + receptor activates a segment of DNA.

4 That activation causes a series of events that result in the production of functional proteins, especially actin and myosin.

5 The new proteins give the muscle cell increased size and strength.

CHAPTER TWO

Food Really Is Fuel

Eat and drink wisely because food and fluid intake affect performance, recovery, and adaptation.

Every muscle contraction is ultimately made possible by the sun. That's because every muscle contraction requires energy, and biological energy on Earth originates with the sun. Energy contained in sunlight is captured by plant life on land and in water and converted through photosynthesis into fuel: carbohydrate, protein, and fat. Animals consume plants (and sometimes each other), capturing the energy contained in plant nutrients for conversion into the carbohydrate, protein, and fat needed for animal growth and daily movement. Humans consume plants and animals to capture the carbohydrate, protein, and fat needed for growth and daily movement. As the saying goes, you are what you eat.

From Food to Energy

The energy contained in carbohydrate, fat, and protein form the energy required for all metabolic processes, including muscle contraction. From those food sources, the body creates a useable form of energy molecule, adenosine triphosphate, or ATP (figure 2.1).

Even though the total amount of ATP in the human body is only 100 grams (about 3 oz) at any given time, each day the human body produces the equivalent of roughly half of its body weight in ATP. That fact is clear evidence that even when not exercising, the body needs a lot of ATP. How is all that ATP used?

It should be no surprise that ATP production increases dramatically during exercise. The more intense the exercise, the more ATP muscles have to produce to maintain those contractions. In fact, the body fatigues whenever muscles can no longer produce ATP fast enough to fuel muscle contractions. The body needs ATP for functions beyond muscle contraction, but during exercise, muscles are the main consumers of the ATP produced within each muscle cell.

Why not just eat some ATP to maximally fuel muscles for exercise? Unfortunately, that tantalizing proposition doesn't work because, although ATP is a tiny molecule, it's still too large to get across cell membranes. That's actually a good thing because if ATP were able to cross cell membranes, the ATP produced by muscle cells during exercise would leak out

Each muscle cell contains about one billion ATP molecules, all of which will be used and replaced every 2 minutes.

A molecule of ATP consists of an adenosine group and three inorganic phosphates. The high-energy bonds between the inorganic phosphates store a lot of energy.

When a cell needs energy, the enzyme ATPase breaks one of the phosphates from ATP, releasing energy that can be used by the cell. An ADP molecule — adenosine diphosphate — and an inorganic phosphate molecule are left over.

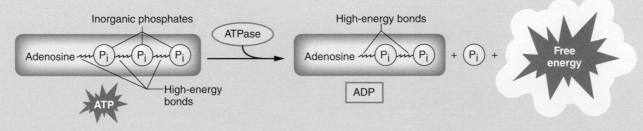

I FIGURE 2.1 Adenosine triphosphate (ATP) molecule.

of the cells, robbing the cells of the energy needed for muscle contraction. Another problem with ingesting ATP is that most of it would be digested in the stomach and small intestine, so only the bits and pieces of ATP molecules would be absorbed. (By the way, the same limitations exist for eating the enzymes necessary to produce ATP; they also are digested into their constituent amino acids before being absorbed across the cells of the small intestine into the bloodstream.)

How the Body Uses ATP

- Powering muscle contraction
- Pumping nutrients across cell membranes
- Pumping calcium back into the sarcoplasmic reticulum in muscles
- Nerve conduction
- Synthesizing proteins in all cells
- Absorbing nutrients in the intestine

Although macronutrients (carbohydrate, fat, and protein) can be broken down to form ATP, they are also used by the body in other ways. All the macronutrients consumed on a daily basis meet one of these fates:

Carbohydrate is broken down (oxidized) to produce ATP energy, stored as glycogen inside cells to meet future energy needs, or used as part of the structure of other molecules (glycoproteins are one example).

Fat (fatty acids to be precise) can be broken down inside cells to produce ATP energy, stored as triglycerides inside fat cells (adipocytes) as well as other cells, or used in various structural ways, often as the primary component of cell membranes.

Protein (actually the amino acids that constitute proteins) is primarily used to form various types of proteins throughout the body. But under some circumstances it can also be broken down to produce ATP energy or converted into fatty acids or glucose. The body is programmed to minimize the use of proteins as energy or for conversion to fatty acids or glucose because protein is a precious commodity. Unlike fat and glucose, excess protein is not stored in the body, so it tries to protect the protein it has. (See figure 2.2.)

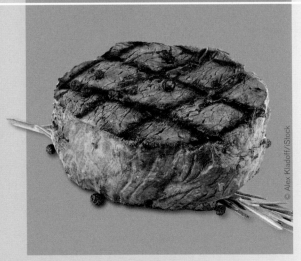

How Do Nutrients Fuel Muscle?

The ATP that muscles need for sustaining contractions and performing many other simultaneous functions in the muscle cell is produced by three sources, all of which are constantly producing ATP.

❶ The breakdown of phosphocreatine (PCr)

❷ The breakdown of carbohydrate (glucose)

❸ The breakdown of fat (fatty acids)

Protein is not a major source of ATP, and that's a very good thing! If protein were used to produce ATP, muscle cells would constantly be breaking down structural and contractile proteins to produce ATP. Fortunately, muscle cells are well designed to break down (oxidize) carbohydrate and fat to produce ATP, sparing the proteins that are so important for other functions inside the cell.

The human body contains 200,000 types of protein.

FIGURE 2.2 Breakdown of carbohydrate, fat, and protein.

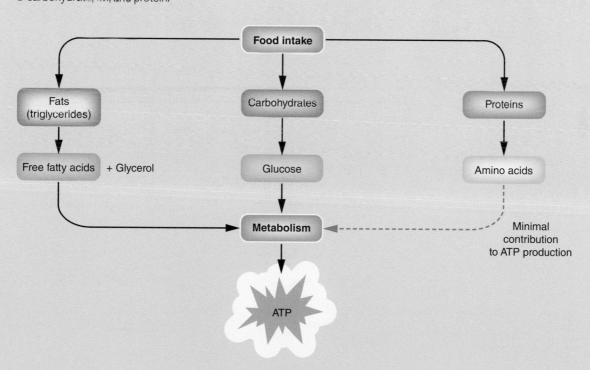

Energy Systems

As you may know, muscle cells can rely on three ways (systems) to produce the ATP needed for muscle contraction. (See figure 2.3.) What is also important to remember is that those energy systems are constantly producing ATP at all times. The intensity of exercise determines which energy system produces most of the ATP at any given time.

FIGURE 2.3 In muscle cells, ATP can be produced by the phosphocreatine (PCr) system, anaerobic glycolysis, the citric acid cycle (also known as the Krebs cycle or the tricarboxylic acid [TCA] cycle), and the electron transport chain. All of these energy-producing systems work simultaneously and in coordination with one another.

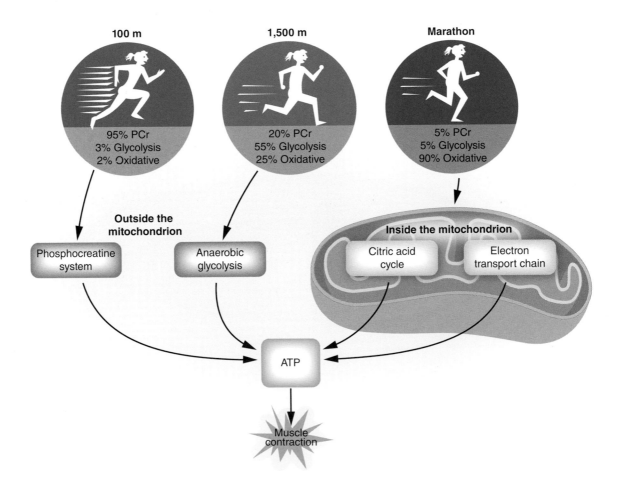

For example, during explosive movements of short duration, such as a 100-meter sprint on the track, most ATP is produced by the phosphocreatine (PCr) system, while the breakdown of carbohydrate and fat contributes a comparatively small amount of ATP. The breakdown of phosphocreatine is a simple reaction requiring only one quick step to produce an ATP molecule. Unfortunately, the PCr content of muscle is fairly small, so the PCr system can produce ATP for only short durations before PCr content falls to low levels.

Anaerobic glycolysis can also produce ATP quickly by breaking down (oxidizing) glucose from the blood and from muscle glycogen stores. (Glycogen is simply a storage form for glucose that enables cells to keep a ready supply of carbohydrate energy close at hand.) The term *anaerobic* is used because this process does not require oxygen. Glycolysis occurs in the sarcoplasm (cytoplasm) of muscle cells so that the ATP produced can be easily used for muscle contraction. Deposits of glycogen are also nearby. Glycolysis is a series of reactions that break glucose molecules in half, capturing the released energy as ATP. The result of breaking glucose in half is two pyruvate molecules (also referred to as pyruvic acid). Pyruvate molecules can quickly be transformed into lactate (lactic acid) molecules during intense exercise or can enter the mitochondria and contribute to the aerobic production of ATP in the citric acid cycle.

Aerobic production of ATP occurs in the many mitochondria in muscle cells. The citric acid cycle (also referred to as the Krebs cycle or the tricarboxylic acid cycle) breaks down pyruvate molecules to produce ATP, carbon dioxide (CO_2), and hydrogen ions (H^+). The ATP is shuttled out of the mitochondria and made available for muscle contraction. The CO_2 diffuses out of the muscle cells into the bloodstream, where it is transported to the lungs to be exhaled with each breath, a process detailed in chapter 3. The H^+ ions are used in the electron transport chain to produce large quantities of ATP along with water and heat. The electron transport chain is where the oxygen (O_2) breathed is used by the muscle cell; two H^+ combine with one O to form water, H_2O. The complete oxidation of glucose through glycolysis followed by the citric acid cycle and electron transport chain produces 32 or 33 ATP (depending on whether the original source is muscle glycogen or blood glucose).

Vitamins and minerals play important roles in all processes leading up to ATP production.

Muscle cells also use fat to produce ATP energy. Fat is stored in small quantities inside muscle cells as intramuscular triglycerides and in large amounts in fat cells (adipocytes). Triglycerides are broken down into fatty acids, and those fatty acids can be transported in the blood to muscles and other cells to produce ATP. Fatty acids are long chains of carbon molecules along with many hydrogen molecules and a few oxygen molecules. Once the fatty acids are cleaved into two-carbon molecules, those small pieces enter the citric acid cycle following the same path as pyruvate molecules. Because fatty acids are much larger than glucose or pyruvate, each fatty acid produces almost 4 times as much ATP energy. For example, oxidation of one molecule of the fatty acid palmitate produces 129 ATP. Unfortunately, fatty acids cannot be broken down very rapidly. As a result, ATP production from fat is important during endurance exercise (and at rest) but less important during shorter-duration, more intense exercise that requires rapid production of ATP. However, fatty acids are still broken down during intense exercise and contribute a small amount of ATP to power muscle contractions.

Glucose: The Body's Most Important Fuel

Phosphocreatine stores are limited and fatty acids are oxidized slowly, but carbohydrate (glucose) can be oxidized quickly by anaerobic glycolysis and aerobically in the citric acid cycle to keep up with the demands for ATP during all exercise that lasts more than 10 seconds. For that reason, carbohydrate is the most important fuel for muscle cells. *Carbohydrate* is a catch-all term that refers to a lot of molecules with similar characteristics, from simple sugar such as glucose (blood sugar), fructose (fruit sugar), and sucrose (table sugar) to more complex forms of carbohydrate such as starch and fiber.

Glucose is the simple sugar—a *monosaccharide*—that the cells rely on every minute of every day to produce ATP. In fact, under normal circumstances the brain and nerves use only glucose as fuel to produce ATP, a reliance that becomes obvious whenever blood sugar level falls too low. Figure 2.4 shows the structure of glucose and some other forms of simple carbohydrate.

Two monosaccharide sugars combined form a *disaccharide*. When simple sugars are combined in chains longer than two sugars, the resulting molecules are referred to as *oligosaccharides*. For example, a common oligosaccharide used in sports foods and beverages is maltodextrin, chains of 3 to 10 glucose molecules. Disaccharides and oligosaccharides are quickly digested into their component monosaccharides by digestive enzymes in the small intestine. The resulting glucose, fructose, and galactose are absorbed through the cells of the small intestine and released into the bloodstream. Very few cells have the enzymes needed for using fructose and galactose, but the liver converts those

The brain relies solely on glucose for energy. Each day, your brain consumes roughly 130 grams of glucose.

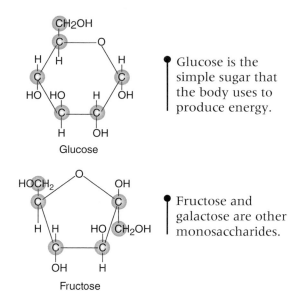

● Glucose is the simple sugar that the body uses to produce energy.

● Fructose and galactose are other monosaccharides.

● Sucrose, the carbohydrate that makes up table sugar (a disaccharide), is formed when fructose and glucose bond together. Similarly, lactose, a sugar found in milk, is formed when glucose and galactose share a bond. Maltose is the combination of two glucose molecules.

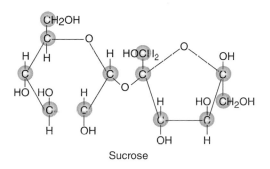

FIGURE 2.4 All monosaccharides have the same chemical makeup—$C_6H_{12}O_6$—but different molecular structures.

During intense exercise, muscles use more than 2 grams of glucose per minute, but muscles are only capable of using a little more than 1 gram of glucose per minute from carbohydrate ingested during exercise.

two sugars into glucose that the liver can store as glycogen or release into the bloodstream for use by other cells.

Starches and fibers (and glycogen) are *polysaccharides* composed of thousands of glucose molecules arranged in long branched chains. Starches can be broken down into glucose, a digestive process that starts with enzymes in the mouth and finishes inside the small intestine. These enzymes break large starch molecules into smaller pieces that can be further broken apart by other enzymes into monosaccharides. With fibers such as cellulose, the bonds that hold the glucose molecules together cannot be broken apart; therefore, fibers are not digested and absorbed. Interestingly, many of the bacteria that live in the large intestine can consume fibers to produce the ATP they need to survive. The activity of those bacteria contributes to overall health.

Keep in mind that regardless of the form of carbohydrate you ingest, glucose is the final product used by your body. (See figure 2.5.) For instance, if you consume a breakfast of orange juice, cereal, and whole-grain toast, the monosaccharides, disaccharides, oligosaccharides, and polysaccharides in those foods all end up as glucose in your body. The speed at which carbohydrate enters the bloodstream and is made available to muscle and other tissues depends in part on how rapidly a meal or snack exits the stomach into the small intestine, where digestion and absorption occur. The more Calories you put into the stomach, the slower that food empties into the small intestine.

Whenever you consume sports drinks, carbohydrate gels, and nutrition bars during exercise, the carbohydrate is quickly absorbed and converted into glucose that muscle cells can extract from the bloodstream and metabolize for ATP. In fact, during intense exercise, muscles can use more than 1 gram per minute from carbohydrate ingested during exercise. That extra energy helps muscle maintain a high rate of carbohydrate oxidation, improving performance capacity.

What About Fat and Protein?

A balanced diet contains a variety of foods and therefore a variety of carbohydrate, fat, and protein. Figure 2.6 maps out some of the types of fat. Fat is consumed either as individual fatty acids or as triglycerides (three fatty acids connected to one glycerol molecule). Enzymes in the small intestine break apart the triglycerides so that individual fatty acids can be absorbed and distributed in the bloodstream to cells throughout the body (figure 2.7). Cells take up fatty acids for use as part of the cell's membrane, as the building blocks for other molecules, or to break down to form ATP.

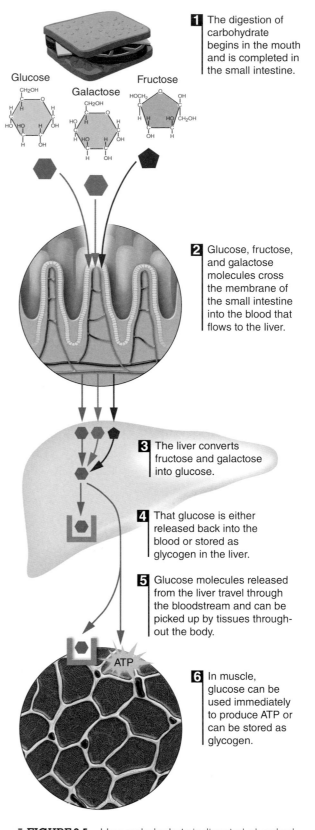

1 The digestion of carbohydrate begins in the mouth and is completed in the small intestine.

2 Glucose, fructose, and galactose molecules cross the membrane of the small intestine into the blood that flows to the liver.

3 The liver converts fructose and galactose into glucose.

4 That glucose is either released back into the blood or stored as glycogen in the liver.

5 Glucose molecules released from the liver travel through the bloodstream and can be picked up by tissues throughout the body.

6 In muscle, glucose can be used immediately to produce ATP or can be stored as glycogen.

FIGURE 2.5 How carbohydrate is digested, absorbed, and used by the body.

Fat in food is in the form of triglycerides, which are simply three fatty acids connected to one glycerol molecule. Triglycerides are the form in which fat is stored by plants and animals, including humans.

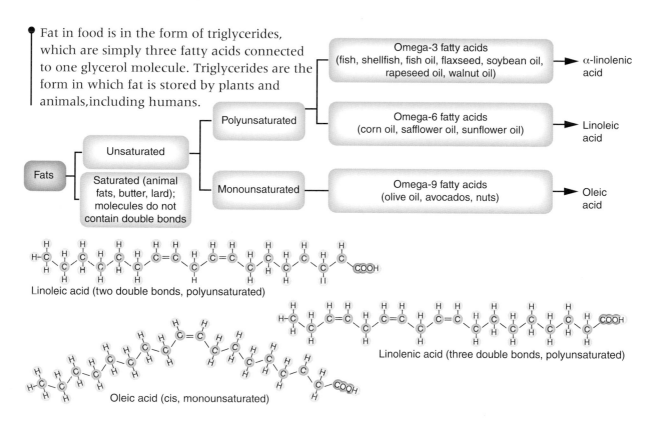

FIGURE 2.6 There are many types of fatty acids that vary in length and in number of oxygen and hydrogen atoms. Muscles can break down any fatty acid to produce ATP.

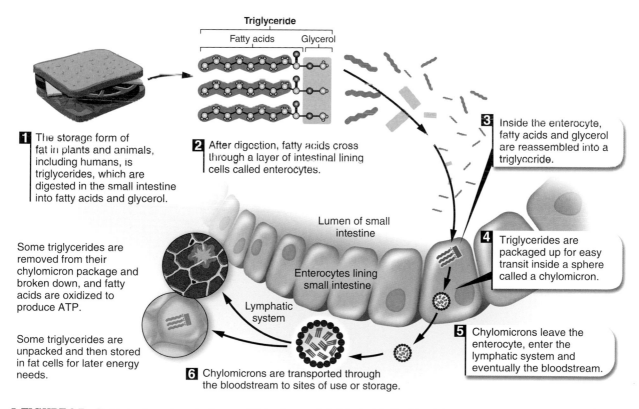

1 The storage form of fat in plants and animals, including humans, is triglycerides, which are digested in the small intestine into fatty acids and glycerol.

2 After digestion, fatty acids cross through a layer of intestinal lining cells called enterocytes.

3 Inside the enterocyte, fatty acids and glycerol are reassembled into a triglyceride.

4 Triglycerides are packaged up for easy transit inside a sphere called a chylomicron.

5 Chylomicrons leave the enterocyte, enter the lymphatic system and eventually the bloodstream.

6 Chylomicrons are transported through the bloodstream to sites of use or storage.

Some triglycerides are removed from their chylomicron package and broken down, and fatty acids are oxidized to produce ATP.

Some triglycerides are unpacked and then stored in fat cells for later energy needs.

FIGURE 2.7 Fat is broken down in the small intestine and distributed in the blood for use as energy or to be stored.

The protein in foods, including meat, fish, dairy products, and beans, is digested with the help of acids and enzymes in the stomach, and enzymes from the small intestine finish the job of breaking proteins into individual amino acids. Of the 20 amino acids that the body needs, 9 have to be supplied by food; the other 11 can be synthesized by the body as needed. Those 9 amino acids are referred to as the *essential amino acids*. (See table 2.1.) When it comes to building and repairing muscle, the essential amino acids are, well, essential. That doesn't mean that essential amino acids are the only amino acids used to build and repair muscle, because all of the amino acids are used to create proteins. But it does mean that the essential amino acids have to be present for protein building to occur. If you don't eat enough essential amino acids, your body scavenges existing proteins, and that is something to avoid. But when it comes to producing ATP inside muscle cells, amino acids are the fuel of *last* choice. After all, why would any cell want to break down its own proteins to make ATP? Doing so would degrade the cell's structure and internal functions. That's why cells rely on glucose and fatty acids, not amino acids, to make ATP. Figure 2.8 shows the pathway of protein breakdown in the body.

The daily protein requirement is estimated to be 0.8 gram per kilogram of body weight per day. At least that's the value for people who aren't very physically active. For athletes and others who exercise more than an hour each day, daily protein needs rise because more protein is needed for growth and repair of muscle cells. Endurance athletes are advised to consume 1.2 to 1.4 grams of protein per kilogram per day (often expressed as g/kg/day). For strength and power athletes, the value is 1.2 to 1.7 g/kg/day (0.5-0.8 g/lb/day). In other words, a 100-pound athlete should consume 50 to 80 grams of protein each day. Even a 300-pound athlete needs only 150 to 240 grams of protein daily. To keep things in perspective, 300 grams of protein

TABLE 2.1 **Essential and Nonessential Amino Acids**

Essential	Nonessential
Isoleucine	Alanine
Leucine	Arginine
Lysine	Asparagine
Methionine	Aspartic acid
Phenylalanine	Cysteine
Threonine	Glutamic acid
Tryptophan	Glutamine
Valine	Glycine
Histidine (children)*	Proline
	Serine
	Tyrosine
	Histidine (adult)*

*Histidine is not synthesized in infants and young children, so it is an essential amino acid for children but not for adults.

About 100 million protein molecules are in each cell, and each cell contains at least 20,000 types of proteins.

is roughly 10 ounces, the amount in one medium-sized steak. Ingesting the recommended amount of protein is easy for any athlete who consumes a balanced diet. In other words, protein powders and amino acid supplements usually aren't needed. However, for athletes on restricted diets or those who have poor eating habits, a protein supplement or shake can help ensure adequate protein intake at no risk to health.

Research shows that consuming protein after exercise can boost muscle protein synthesis, giving athletes a jump start on muscle growth and recovery. Equally interesting and of great practical value is that not much protein is needed. It takes only 20 grams of a high-quality protein to maximally boost muscle protein synthesis. In addition, consuming small snacks high in protein every couple hours throughout the day provides a further boost to muscle protein synthesis. Dairy products appear to be particularly effective at boosting muscle protein synthesis because dairy protein is high in essential amino acids, especially the essential amino acid leucine, which is a spark for muscle protein synthesis. This is the reason many sport nutrition experts recommend that athletes consume a large glass of chocolate milk after hard workouts (cow's milk contains 1 gram of protein per fluid ounce, and the sugar in the chocolate helps to replenish carbohydrate).

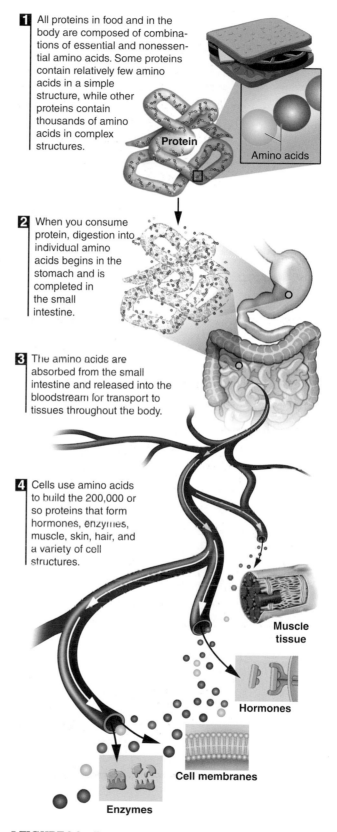

1. All proteins in food and in the body are composed of combinations of essential and nonessential amino acids. Some proteins contain relatively few amino acids in a simple structure, while other proteins contain thousands of amino acids in complex structures.

Protein **Amino acids**

2. When you consume protein, digestion into individual amino acids begins in the stomach and is completed in the small intestine.

3. The amino acids are absorbed from the small intestine and released into the bloodstream for transport to tissues throughout the body.

4. Cells use amino acids to build the 200,000 or so proteins that form hormones, enzymes, muscle, skin, hair, and a variety of cell structures.

Muscle tissue

Hormones

Cell membranes

Enzymes

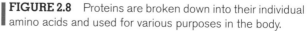

FIGURE 2.8 Proteins are broken down into their individual amino acids and used for various purposes in the body.

Putting It All Together

Figure 2.9 summarizes the paths of carbohydrate, fat, and protein in the body. Carbohydrate, protein, and fat from food provide the ATP energy needed by all cells and are used to repair, replace, and add new cellular structures, such as amino acids from food being used to create new muscle proteins.

As noted earlier, all energy systems continuously produce ATP. The intensity of physical activity determines which energy system is the primary producer of ATP. Under normal circumstances, the body stores lots of usable energy in fat, liver, and muscle cells. Figure 2.10 is a pie chart that depicts the various fuel stores in the body.

FIGURE 2.9   Cellular metabolism results from the breakdown of three fuel substrates provided by the diet. Once each is converted to its usable form, it either circulates in the blood as an available "pool" to be used for metabolism or is stored in the body.

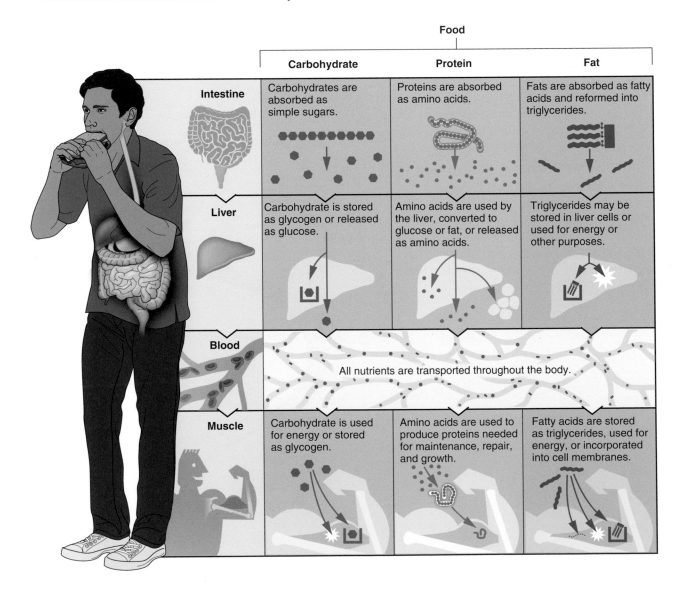

FIGURE 2.10 The body stores fat and carbohydrate energy in fat, liver, and muscle cells.

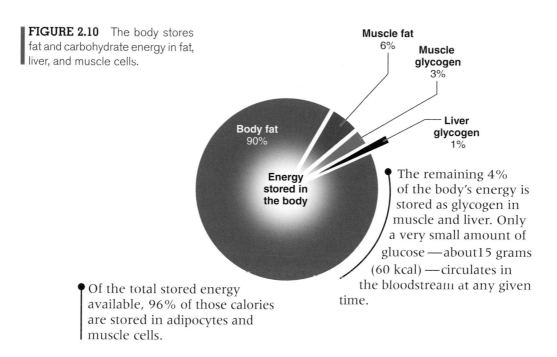

Muscle fat 6%

Muscle glycogen 3%

Liver glycogen 1%

Body fat 90%

Energy stored in the body

The remaining 4% of the body's energy is stored as glycogen in muscle and liver. Only a very small amount of glucose —about 15 grams (60 kcal) —circulates in the bloodstream at any given time.

Of the total stored energy available, 96% of those calories are stored in adipocytes and muscle cells.

Although you can store more than 2,000 Calories of energy as muscle glycogen, fat stores amount to more than 75,000 Calories (in a 140-pound person with 12% body fat), so you're well supplied for low-intensity exercise as long as you can consume enough carbohydrate to maintain blood glucose concentration. During prolonged endurance events such as marathons, Ironman triathlons, and ultraendurance competitions, fatty acids can provide a considerable amount of the needed energy (ATP), reducing the demand on blood glucose and muscle glycogen. Maintaining blood glucose by ingesting sports drinks and consuming carbohydrate-rich snacks (e.g., energy bars, carbohydrate gels, pretzels, fruit) ensures that the brain and nerves have a constant supply of glucose from the blood.

Dietary Supplements and Energy

Energy drinks and similar supplements are popular products because having more energy throughout the day is an appealing concept, especially when it comes time to train or compete. Most energy drinks and supplements do contain energy in the form of carbohydrate, but they also contain varying amounts of caffeine (a stimulant to the central nervous system) as well as other ingredients with stimulant properties such as synephrine, guarana, yohimbe, and green tea extract. Ingesting caffeine does increase alertness and mental focus and can improve endurance performance. Energy drinks typically contain 160 to 260 milligrams of caffeine in 16 ounces (475 ml). By comparison, 16 ounces of coffee contains 200 to 300 milligrams of caffeine, and colas have roughly 70 to 120 milligrams of caffeine per 16 ounces. As with everything in the diet, energy drinks can be consumed safely in moderation. For example, for athletes and clients who enjoy energy drinks, consuming one 16-ounce energy drink 45 to 60 minutes before training or competition may provide enough caffeine to improve performance. Aside from the caffeine and carbohydrate in energy drinks, there is no good scientific evidence that other common ingredients such as taurine and glucuronolactone provide any measurable benefits.

Take a quick look at figure 2.11 and you'll see that the rate at which each energy system can produce ATP varies widely, as does the amount of ATP each system can produce. The PCr system can produce ATP quickly but can't produce much of it. On the other end of the ATP-producing spectrum, fat oxidation produces ATP slowly but can produce it for a long time. The varying capacities for ATP production ensures that cells usually get the ATP they need. One exception is during intense exercise, when the energy systems can't produce ATP fast enough to fuel muscle contraction, a topic covered in chapter 4. Table 2.2 summarizes the characteristics of the various energy systems.

Regular physical exercise increases muscles' capacity to use fat and carbohydrate to produce ATP because exercise prompts muscles to increase the signaling pathways, enzymes, and mitochondria responsible for ATP production. A proper diet, including adequate hydration before, during, and after exercise, provides the macro- and micronutrients that all cells require to generate the ATP needed for the function, repair, and growth of cells.

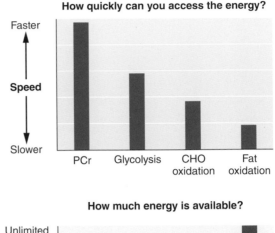

How quickly can you access the energy?

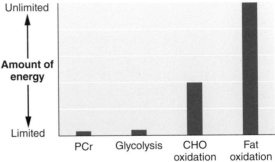

How much energy is available?

FIGURE 2.11 The rate of energy production and the amount of energy that can be produced vary inversely.

Adapted from Kenney, Wilmore, and Costill 2015, *Physiology of sport and exercise*, 6th ed. (Champaign, IL: Human Kinetics), 68.

TABLE 2.2 **Characteristics of the Various Energy Supply Systems**

Energy system	Oxygen necessary?	Overall chemical reaction	Relative rate of ATP formed per second	ATP formed per molecule of substrate	Available capacity
ATP-PCr	No	PCr to Cr	10	1	<15 sec
Glycolysis	No	Glucose or glycogen to lactate	5	2-3	~1 min
Oxidative (from carbohydrate)	Yes	Glucose or glycogen to CO_2 and H_2O	2.5	36-39	~90 min
Oxidative (from fat)	Yes	FFA or triglycerides to CO_2 and H_2O	1.5	>100	Days

Courtesy of Dr. Martin Gibala, McMaster University, Hamilton, Ontario, Canada.

What About Vitamins and Minerals?

Vitamins are essential nutrients the body cannot make, so there's no doubt that you need to consume vitamins on a daily basis to ensure that all cells are supplied with the substances needed for metabolism—not just energy metabolism but metabolism of all sorts. Even though the body contains roughly 10 thousand trillion cells, each cell needs only a tiny amount of vitamins to operate efficiently. Consuming more vitamins than a cell can use is like having more hammers on a construction site than the workers can use. The extras do no good.

Some vitamins are soluble in water, others in fat. That distinction is important because fat-soluble vitamins (A, D, E, K) are stored and used in liver and fat, whereas water-soluble vitamins (B vitamins, C) are used in the watery environments inside muscle and other cells. All are needed in small amounts to supply cells with the vitamins to support bodily functions. Figure 2.12 is an overview of some of the functions of vitamins and minerals.

Some enzymes can perform 1,000 functions per second.

FIGURE 2.12 Some of the functions of vitamins and minerals in the body.

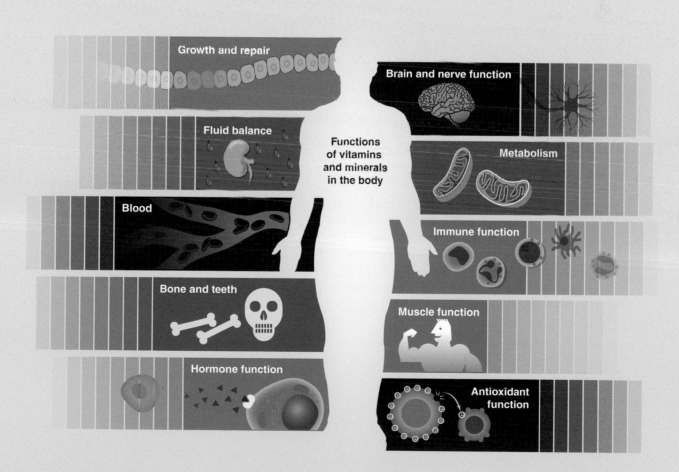

Growth and repair

Brain and nerve function

Fluid balance

Metabolism

Functions of vitamins and minerals in the body

Blood

Immune function

Bone and teeth

Muscle function

Hormone function

Antioxidant function

Vitamins play an important role

in energy metabolism. That's especially true of the B vitamins because they act as cofactors in a variety of enzymatic reactions in the steps that break down glucose and fatty acids. Once each of the muscle cells has enough vitamins to act as cofactors, the body has no choice but to excrete extra vitamins in the urine. Because enzymes, like all other proteins in the body, break down and are replaced on an ongoing basis, you need to consume small amounts of vitamins every day to ensure that the cells have a steady supply. Table 2.3 lists the recommended daily intakes for important vitamins and minerals. That's easily accomplished with a balanced diet. But, as with protein needs, if athletes have poor dietary habits or are on restricted diets, a low-dose multivitamin and mineral supplement can be a low-cost, low-risk way to ensure adequate intake.

Speaking of minerals, as with vitamins, the body needs a small supply of minerals each day because minerals are lost in urine and sweat and relies on food to replace those minerals. Minerals play a variety of roles in the body (figure 2.12). Some minerals are involved in ATP production, while others are involved in nerve conduction, bone formation, red blood cell production, and so on. Although all cells need minerals, daily need is small and can easily be met by consuming a balanced diet, especially if you're not physically active. Table 2.3 gives general guidelines for mineral intake, but the amount of minerals needed in the diet varies widely because mineral use and loss vary widely. Whenever you sweat, mineral loss is increased because sweat contains minerals such as sodium, chloride, potassium, calcium, and magnesium. (Minerals are also referred to as electrolytes because each carries either a positive or negative charge.) With some athletes, daily sweat loss can be greater than 8 liters, so daily mineral loss will also be high. In most cases, eating enough food energy (Calories) supplies more than enough minerals to replace sweat mineral losses, so mineral deficiencies are very rare. One possible exception to that statement is the calcium needs of female athletes. Because many females do not consume enough calcium-rich foods to meet the recommendations for daily calcium intake (1,000 to 1,300 mg), and because calcium is lost in sweat, female athletes should be educated on consuming adequate calcium on a daily basis.

TABLE 2.3 Recommended Dietary Allowance of Vitamins and Minerals

Vitamin or mineral	Adult RDA/AI
VITAMINS	
A	Women: 700 mcg Men: 900 mcg
B_1 (thiamin)	Women: 1.1 mg Men: 1.2 mg
B_2 (riboflavin)	Women: 1.1 mg Men: 1.3 mg
B_3 (niacin)	35 mg
B_6 (pyridoxine)	1.3 mg
B_{12} (cobalamin)	2.4 mcg
C (ascorbic acid)	Women: 75 mg Men: 90 mg
D (cholecalciferol)	600 IU
E (tocopherols)	15 mg
K (phylloquinone)	Women: 90 mcg Men: 120 mcg
Biotin	30 mcg
Folate	400 mcg
Pantothenic acid	5 mg
MINERALS	
Calcium	1,300 mg
Chloride	2,300 mg
Copper	0.9 mg
Fluoride	
Iodine	0.15 mg
Iron	18 mg
Magnesium	420 mg
Manganese	2.3 mg
Molybdenum	0.045 mg
Phosphorous	700 mg
Potassium	4,700 mg
Selenium	0.055 mg
Sodium	1,500 mg
Zinc	1 mg

Water Is a Nutrient, Too

For anyone who is physically active, water is the most important nutrient. Water is not only the most biologically active molecule in the body, but it is also the nutrient lost in the greatest amount on a daily basis. Even on days when you don't produce even a drop of sweat, you still need to drink at least 2 liters of fluid. In fact, the U.S. Institute of Medicine recommends a daily fluid intake of 2.7 liters for females and 3.7 liters for males. These values are estimates of the volumes of fluid American adults should consume each day, but for anyone who breaks a sweat, fluid needs can be much higher. For example, most people are capable of losing 500 to 1,000 milliliters (roughly 16-32 oz) of sweat per hour of exercise. A woman who does a hard 2-hour workout and loses 1.5 liters of sweat may have a daily fluid requirement in excess of 4 liters. That's a lot of fluid! Roughly 65% of body weight is plain old water (less as body fat increases), and that figure alone gives a quick indication of how important water molecules must be for bodily functions. (See figure 2.13.)

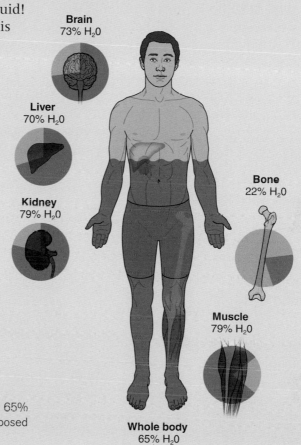

Brain
73% H_2O

Liver
70% H_2O

Kidney
79% H_2O

Bone
22% H_2O

Muscle
79% H_2O

Whole body
65% H_2O

FIGURE 2.13 The human body is about 65% water by weight, but some tissues are composed of even more water.

Drinking for Hydration

Women

2.7 liters per day = 90 ounces per day

20% from food = 18 ounces

80% from beverages = 72 ounces

Drink at least 16 ounces with each meal.

Drink at least 8 ounces between meals.

Drink whenever sweaty.

Men

3.7 liters per day = 125 ounces per day

20% from food = 25 ounces

80% from beverages = 100 ounces

Drink at least 24 ounces with each meal.

Drink at least 10 ounces between meals.

Drink whenever sweaty.

The body's fluid-regulatory mechanisms are pretty good at maintaining proper hydration levels during rest so that at the end of each day, you have much the same volume of water in your body as you had at the start of the day. That's really no small task because, while you are constantly losing fluid, you only periodically drink it. The kidneys continuously produce urine, your skin constantly leaks small quantities of water, and each breath you exhale contains water molecules from the lungs. Those three avenues of fluid loss add up to the recommended 2.7 and 3.7 liters per day. If you eat a diet that contains fruits and vegetables, you can ingest about 20% of daily fluid needs from food. The remaining 80% you have to drink. The good news is that virtually all beverages count for meeting daily hydration needs (shots of alcohol excluded). With easy access to water, milk, fruit juices, coffee, tea, soft drinks, flavored waters, and sports drinks, you shouldn't have any difficulty staying hydrated. Yet dehydration is still common, especially among those who are physically active. That's because your thirst mechanism is designed to protect you against severe dehydration, not mild dehydration. Fortunately, most fluid intake occurs spontaneously with meals or on other occasions (in meetings or at parties, for example) where drinking occurs in the absence of thirst.

Because even a little dehydration impairs a variety of physiological responses as well as physical and even mental performance, it's always better to be well hydrated than dehydrated. For that reason, the best advice is to drink enough fluid (water or sports drinks) during physical activity to minimize loss of body weight. Weight loss during exercise is virtually all sweat loss, so drinking enough to minimize that loss maintains good hydration and provides the fluid needed to maintain blood volume. When you allow yourself to

Water Is Constantly Lost From the Body During Rest

- Kidneys are constantly producing urine.
- Water molecules constantly seep through the skin in small quantities.
- Every exhalation is saturated with water molecules.
- Feces accounts for a few ounces of water loss each day.

become dehydrated, blood volume shrinks, reducing blood flow to muscles and skin (for heat loss) and causing other negative physiological responses. The simple solution is to drink enough to stay well hydrated (minimize weight loss). That's why it's important to periodically weigh yourself before and after workouts to see if your hydration habits are keeping pace with your sweat loss.

The daily requirement for water also varies widely not only from person to person but also from day to day for the same person. A small, sedentary person living in a cool environment will need less water than a larger, physically active person living in a warm environment. And you need less water on days you don't exercise than on days you do. Your body regulates fluid intake primarily by altering the sensation of thirst and kidney function. If you consume too much fluid, thirst diminishes and the kidneys increase urine production. On those occasions when you don't drink enough, thirst is increased and kidneys reduce urine production.

Most of the fluid consumed on a daily basis comes from beverages, and a smaller amount (about 20%) comes from food. The U.S. Institute of Medicine estimates that adult men should consume 125 ounces (3.7 L) of water each day (100 oz from beverages, 25 oz from foods). For adult women, the value drops to 90 ounces per day (2.7 L; 74 oz from beverages; 16 oz from foods). Those values are only estimates of the daily requirements for most adults. Athletes, workers, soldiers— all who work up a sweat—have an increased daily requirement of water that will likely exceed those values. In fact, some people may need to drink 2 gallons or more each day (7.5 L) simply because they sweat a lot.

Negative Response to Dehydration

- Reduced blood volume
- Reduced stroke volume
- Increased heart rate
- Reduced cardiac output
- Reduced muscle blood flow
- Reduced skin blood flow
- Increased plasma osmolality
- Reduced sweat rate
- Increased body temperature
- Impaired attention and focus
- Impaired endurance performance

When sweat losses are very high, as can be the case during ultramarathons, Ironman-distance triathlons, and two-a-day practices, a lot of sodium is lost from the body. Under those circumstances, drinking large volumes of plain water will cause the sodium level of the blood to drop below normal, a condition known as hyponatremia. The same thing can happen if a resting person drinks a large volume of water quickly. Because you can drink faster than your kidneys can produce urine, the blood sodium level is temporarily diluted. Usually this is not a problem and blood sodium returns to normal. But when the drop in blood sodium is large, swelling of the brain occurs, a condition that can lead to seizures, coma, and death. Exercise-associated hyponatremia is not common, but all sport health professionals should be aware of the possibility and educate physically active people to drink enough fluid to minimize weight loss but avoid overdrinking.

CHAPTER THREE

Muscles Need Oxygen

Aerobic exercise requires oxygen that the heart, lungs, blood, and vasculature are well designed to deliver.

Oxygen is the third-most abundant element in the universe (hydrogen and helium are first and second). In fact, oxygen makes up most of body mass because the human body is mostly water—H_2O—and because oxygen is part of protein, fat, carbohydrate, and many other molecules in the body.

Humans rely on oxygen for the unending production of the ATP molecules, which are essential for cell functions, including muscle contractions. Oxygen in the air is continuously replenished by oxygen released from plants as a by-product of photosynthesis, the process plants use to produce ATP.

The air you breathe is 21% oxygen (O_2), 20.93%, to be precise. The rest (76%) is nitrogen (N_2) with a pinch (0.04%) of carbon dioxide (CO_2). At sea level, the atmospheric pressure ensures that lungs are exposed to enough O_2 molecules with each inhalation that breathing is easy, especially at rest. At altitude, the lower partial pressure of oxygen in the air impairs endurance performance because it limits the amount of oxygen that can be delivered to muscles. But on Mt. Everest, where the atmospheric pressure is only 33% of that at sea level, the O_2 molecules are spread so far apart that it's difficult to catch a breath, even at rest. The air at the peak of Mt. Everest still contains 21% oxygen, but the atmospheric pressure is low because at 29,029 feet (8,848 m), there is much less air above to create pressure. As a result, breathing has to be very rapid to introduce enough oxygen into the lungs to satisfy even the low metabolic needs at rest. This simple fact is why most mountaineers rely on supplemental oxygen at very high altitudes.

©technotr/iStock

How Does Oxygen Get to Muscles?

The human body is obviously well equipped to extract oxygen from inhaled air and deliver that oxygen to all cells in the body, including muscles. That process is actually very simple in concept, even though it's quite complicated in detail.

Lungs allow oxygen from inhaled air to pass across the very thin membranes in the depths of the lungs and enter the bloodstream. At the same time, carbon dioxide that was produced by muscles and other cells leaves the blood, passing across the lung membranes to be exhaled from the body. This exchange is illustrated in figure 3.1.

Some of the oxygen in inhaled air passes across the lungs into the blood. At the same time, carbon dioxide is released from the blood and enters the lungs to be exhaled. The movement of those two gases—O_2 and CO_2—depends on their concentrations and their diffusion coefficients. The diffusion coefficient is a measure of how quickly a substance tends to move across a membrane like the lining of the lung alveoli. For example, even though CO_2 is in low concentration in the blood flowing through the lungs, it moves easily from the blood into the lungs because CO_2 has a high diffusion coefficient, 20 times greater than O_2 has.

Oxygen is so critical to survival that, even at the cellular level, all nucleated cells in the body can sense oxygen.

FIGURE 3.1 The exchange of oxygen and carbon dioxide at the lungs. Oxygen binds to hemoglobin in the blood. Iron is an important part of each hemoglobin molecule.

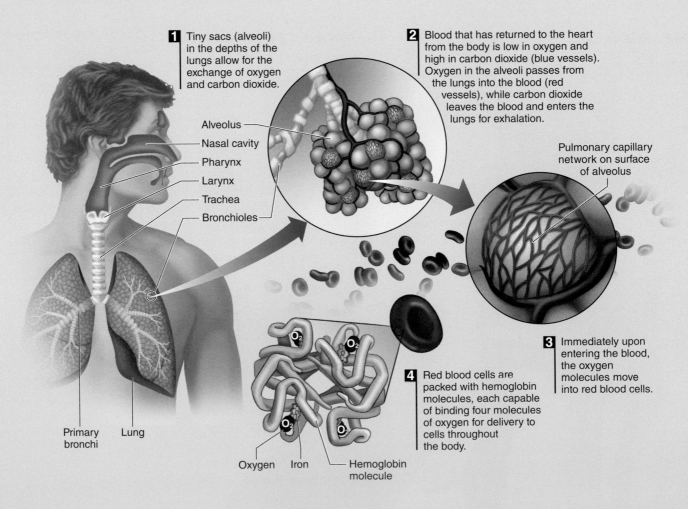

1 Tiny sacs (alveoli) in the depths of the lungs allow for the exchange of oxygen and carbon dioxide.

2 Blood that has returned to the heart from the body is low in oxygen and high in carbon dioxide (blue vessels). Oxygen in the alveoli passes from the lungs into the blood (red vessels), while carbon dioxide leaves the blood and enters the lungs for exhalation.

Pulmonary capillary network on surface of alveolus

Alveolus
Nasal cavity
Pharynx
Larynx
Trachea
Bronchioles

3 Immediately upon entering the blood, the oxygen molecules move into red blood cells.

4 Red blood cells are packed with hemoglobin molecules, each capable of binding four molecules of oxygen for delivery to cells throughout the body.

Primary bronchi   Lung

Oxygen   Iron   Hemoglobin molecule

When oxygenated blood reaches muscle cells, the bond between oxygen and hemoglobin molecules loosens. When the red blood cells pass single file through the tiny capillaries that surround muscle cells (figure 3.2), oxygen molecules are released from hemoglobin and diffuse into the muscle cells. The carbon dioxide produced by the muscle cells diffuses into the bloodstream not as CO_2 but as bicarbonate ion (HCO_3^-) that is converted back into CO_2 in the lungs, where it is exhaled.

Once inside muscle cells, the oxygen can either bind to *myoglobin* (a protein like hemoglobin that enables muscle cells to store a small amount of oxygen) or enter the mitochondria to be used in the electron transport chain to accept the H^+ ions produced by the oxidation of carbohydrate and fat. Before binding with oxygen to form H_2O, the H^+ ions are used in the electron transport chain to produce ATP. The complete oxidation of carbohydrate and fat produces ATP, H_2O, CO_2, and heat.

The process by which carbohydrate and fat are oxidized to produce ATP is referred to as *internal respiration* because it occurs inside cells. The delivery of oxygen from the lungs to the cells is called *external respiration*.

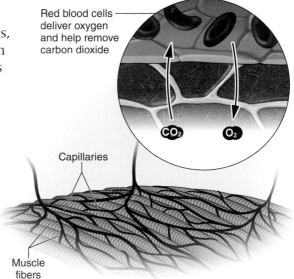

Red blood cells deliver oxygen and help remove carbon dioxide

CO_2 O_2

Capillaries

Muscle fibers

FIGURE 3.2 Muscle cells are supplied by tiny capillaries that deliver oxygen and nutrients and remove waste products such as carbon dioxide and lactic acid.

The Role of Iron in Oxygen Transport

Even though the human body contains only 3 to 4 grams of iron, that small amount plays a variety of important roles. The iron in each hemoglobin molecule binds oxygen for transport; in fact, the color of blood is due in part to those iron molecules. Myoglobin in muscle cells also contains iron molecules; myoglobin serves as a way station for oxygen molecules on their short journey from the red blood cells into the mitochondria. And iron molecules are important for the function of many enzymes.

Iron is a mineral needed in small amounts on a daily basis (8 mg per day). Red meat, beans, fish, and leafy vegetables are good sources of iron. Some female athletes are prone to iron deficiency because of iron loss during menstruation combined with low iron intake in their diets. If iron deficiency becomes severe, anemia (abnormally low hemoglobin level) can result. Iron deficiency and anemia are far more common in females than in males.

Measuring the iron content in blood is not useful in determining a person's iron status, but other measures such as plasma ferritin (the storage form of iron) are used to determine whether someone is iron deficient. If iron stores become too low, the bone marrow has a difficult time maintaining normal hemoglobin production, and iron-deficiency anemia can result. It is possible for athletes to have iron deficiency without anemia; some estimates indicate that 20% to 25% of female athletes are iron deficient (below-normal plasma ferritin levels). Whether or not performance is adversely affected by iron deficiency is a matter of debate, but there is no doubt that iron deficiency is abnormal and should be addressed through changes in diet and perhaps daily intake of an iron supplement.

Reference: Rowland, T. (2012). Iron deficiency in athletes. *American Journal of Lifestyle Medicine, 6*(4):319-327.

As you become more aerobically fit, your capacity to deliver oxygenated blood to active skeletal muscle cells increases. Evidence of that increase is seen as an increased maximal oxygen consumption ($\dot{V}O_{2max}$), which is measured by a laboratory test that requires participants to exercise at increasing workloads to exhaustion (more about this later). Lung function does not change much as the result of improved fitness, but heart function does, and the most important change is an increase in *cardiac output*. In other words, the heart is capable of pumping more blood each minute. Improved fitness also causes blood volume to increase, supporting increased cardiac output. And muscle cells increase their capacity to use oxygen. All of these changes and more enable the increase in $\dot{V}O_{2max}$ and improved aerobic performance. Figure 3.3 is an overview of how lungs, heart, blood, and vasculature work together to deliver oxygen and remove carbon dioxide from all cells.

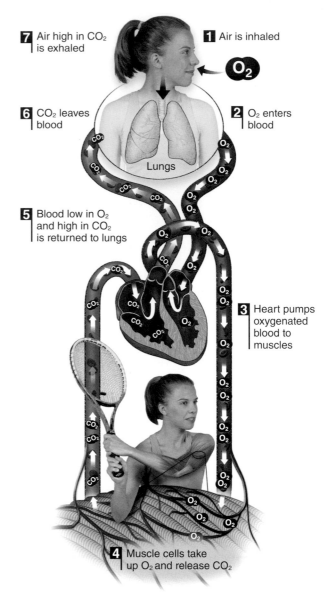

7 Air high in CO_2 is exhaled

1 Air is inhaled

O_2

6 CO_2 leaves blood

2 O_2 enters blood

Lungs

5 Blood low in O_2 and high in CO_2 is returned to lungs

3 Heart pumps oxygenated blood to muscles

4 Muscle cells take up O_2 and release CO_2

FIGURE 3.3 All types of exercise rely on the aerobic production of ATP. The heart, lungs, blood, and vasculature work together to deliver oxygen and remove carbon dioxide.

The body actually has two pumps that move blood to and from the heart. The heart itself is the most obvious pump, but the contraction of skeletal muscles is the second pump that ensures that blood is pushed back to the heart.

How Does Oxygen Use Relate to Fitness and Energy Expenditure?

The body's capacity to use oxygen is a measure of health and fitness. Elite endurance athletes have a large capacity to use oxygen, and that is reflected in their very high maximal oxygen consumption values. At the other end of the spectrum are those with poor physical fitness, who have very low $\dot{V}O_{2max}$ values.

Oxygen consumption measurement is used to determine how much oxygen a person is using each minute. Oxygen consumption can be measured while a person is resting as well as during various types, intensities, and durations of exercise. Not only is *maximal* oxygen consumption an indication of aerobic fitness, oxygen consumption measured during an activity allows scientists to calculate the *energy cost* (caloric cost) of that activity (which is why oxygen consumption testing is also referred to as *indirect calorimetry*). Energy cost (also known as *energy expenditure*) is expressed in *kilocalories* (commonly called Calories). For a 154-pound (70 kg) person, the energy cost of running at 7.5 mph is roughly 14 Calories per minute, a value determined by oxygen consumption testing.

Metabolic Rate at Rest and During Exercise

You might have heard someone say, "She's lean because she must have a high metabolic rate." *Metabolic rate* is simply the rate at which the body uses energy. In other words, metabolic rate, energy expenditure, and oxygen consumption can be considered synonyms. You'll also hear other terms such as *resting metabolic rate* (RMR) and *basal metabolic rate* (BMR) used to refer to the energy expenditure at rest. RMR and BMR are measured in slightly different ways, but the values are similar. In both cases, measures of oxygen consumption can be used to estimate resting energy expenditure.

As an example, consider what the BMR might be for a 128-pound (58 kg) woman with 24% body fat. A person of this size and body composition will consume about 250 milliliters (0.25 L) of oxygen every minute at rest. There are 1,440 minutes in a day, so her oxygen consumption would be 0.25 liter per minute × 1,440 minutes per day = 360 liters of oxygen per day. How do 360 liters of oxygen convert to Calories? For that conversion, you need to know that each liter of oxygen is equivalent to 4.8 Calories (under these circumstances). At this point, the math is simple: This woman's BMR is estimated to be 360 liters per day × 4.8 Calories per liter, or 1,728 Calories per day. Now you know the number of Calories this woman must consume to maintain her current body weight. If she is physically active, the energy cost of her daily activity is added to her BMR to estimate her total energy (caloric) needs.

Oxygen consumption—abbreviated as $\dot{V}O_2$—increases whenever the body needs more oxygen to meet its metabolic needs. It should be no surprise that oxygen consumption at rest is low compared to oxygen consumption during any type of physical activity. Oxygen consumption at rest depends mostly on a person's body size (specifically, on fat-free mass and body surface area). In other words, resting oxygen consumption is higher in larger people than in smaller people because larger people have more cells, all of which require oxygen to function. Once we become active, the more intense the activity, the higher the oxygen consumption. Not surprisingly, the higher your heart rate, the higher your oxygen consumption since the heart efficiently pumps the oxygen-containing blood to those active tissues.

You might have heard the term *MET* (for *metabolic equivalent of training*) used to refer to levels of exercise intensity. One MET is roughly the equivalent to the energy (oxygen) cost of sitting quietly, which is 1 Calorie per kilogram of body weight per hour (1 kcal/kg/hr; about 3.5 ml O_2/kg/min). In other words, an activity that requires 5 METs requires 5 times the energy of sitting quietly. (See the sidebar Factors That Affect Resting Metabolic Rate to learn how RMR can vary from the 1.0 kcal/kg/hr value used to establish 1 MET.)

$\dot{V}O_{2max}$ and What It Means

Maximal oxygen consumption ($\dot{V}O_{2max}$) is a measure of the body's maximal capacity to use oxygen. It is measured as milliliters of oxygen used per kilogram of body weight per minute, which may range from less than 20 ml/kg/min in very deconditioned people to over 70 ml/kg/min in elite endurance athletes. During a maximal exercise test, $\dot{V}O_{2max}$ occurs when the amount of oxygen the person is using does not increase any further in response to increasing exercise intensity. As you become more aerobically fit, muscles increase their capacity to use oxygen. That change allows you to exercise at higher intensities without fatiguing. See figure 3.4 for an example of how one person had a 30% increase in $\dot{V}O_{2max}$, from 44 to 57 ml/kg/min, as a result of training. This magnitude of increase in $\dot{V}O_{2max}$ is fairly typical and generally occurs after 2 to 3 months of proper training.

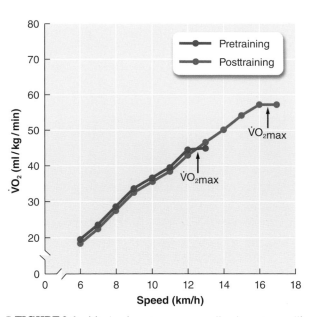

FIGURE 3.4 Maximal oxygen consumption increases with proper training. After 2 to 3 months of training, there are no further increases in $\dot{V}O_{2max}$ in most people.

Reprinted, by permission, from W.L. Kenney, J.H. Willmore, and D.L. Costill, 2015, *Physiology of sport and exercise*, 6th ed. (Champaign, IL: Human Kinetics), 263.

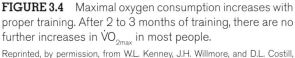

Factors That Affect Resting Metabolic Rate

The largest part of daily energy (caloric) needs is represented by the energy required to fuel resting metabolism. In other words, if all you did was lie in bed all day, all the cells in your body would still break down glucose and fatty acids to produce the ATP required to meet the resting energy needs of each cell. Larger bodies typically need more energy than smaller bodies, so resting metabolic rate (RMR) is understandably greater for larger people than for smaller people.

According to several studies, the RMR for adult men is calculated to be 0.892 kcal/kg/hr; for females, the value is 0.839 kcal/kg/hr. Keep in mind that these values are just good estimates based on a lot of research and take only body weight into consideration. As it turns out, the same research shows that RMR decreases with age as muscle mass decreases, fat mass increases, and the metabolic rate of organs such as the liver and kidneys gradually declines. RMR is also lower in overweight and obese people than it is in normal-weight people. For example, normal-weight women had an RMR of 0.926 kcal/kg/hr compared to 0.721 kcal/kg/hr in obese women. The values were 0.960 and 0.791 in normal-weight and obese men, respectively. Fat is a low-metabolic-rate tissue, while muscle has a comparatively higher resting metabolic rate. For that reason alone, adding muscle and losing fat increase RMR.

The moral of this story is that maintaining a high RMR as you age depends largely on maintaining muscle mass and keeping body fat at normal levels. Happily, both of those goals are attainable through regular physical activity.

Reference: McMurray, R.G., et al. (2014). Examining variations of resting metabolic rate of adults. *Medicine and Science in Sports and Exercise, 46*(7):1352-1358.

After a year or so of training, $\dot{V}O_{2max}$ reaches a plateau and does not increase further. But endurance performance can continue to improve because with training it's possible to exercise at a greater percentage of $\dot{V}O_{2max}$. Imagine that a runner is able to run for an hour at 80% of her $\dot{V}O_{2max}$. With proper training, she might then be able to run for an hour at 86% of her $\dot{V}O_{2max}$, enabling her to run at a faster speed even though her $\dot{V}O_{2max}$ has not increased.

There's no doubt that highly fit people have above-average $\dot{V}O_{2max}$ values. But $\dot{V}O_{2max}$ alone is not a good predictor of endurance performance. Also important to performance is the percentage of $\dot{V}O_{2max}$ that can be sustained over time, as in the previous example. That level of effort is often referred to as the *lactate threshold* (also called *anaerobic threshold* or *ventilatory threshold*). The lactate threshold simply refers to the highest exercise intensity that can be sustained without an accumulation of lactic acid in the bloodstream. Even without the laboratory procedures required for measuring $\dot{V}O_{2max}$ and lactate threshold, experienced athletes know how hard they can push themselves and will lower the intensity before it becomes unsustainable.

Measuring maximal oxygen consumption requires special equipment and experienced staff, so most athletes have to depend on improvements in training and competition as evidence that their aerobic capacity has improved. After all, the result of improved performance is far more important than knowing how much an athlete's maximal oxygen consumption might have improved with training. A variety of aerobic fitness tests have been developed to estimate maximal oxygen consumption. For example, 1.0- or 1.5-mile run times on a track as well as treadmill and cycle ergometer tests can be used to estimate maximal oxygen consumption and assess aerobic fitness.

Elite endurance athletes have very high $\dot{V}O_{2max}$ values: for women, >70 ml/kg/min; for men, >85 ml/kg/min.

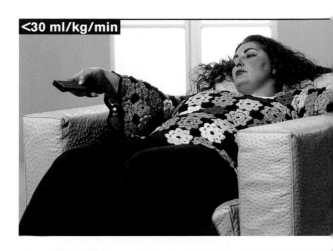

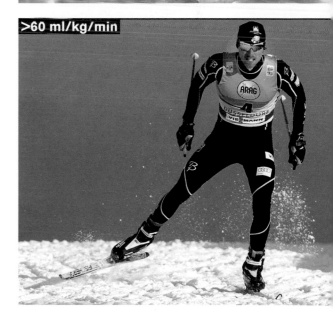

Other Terms You Should Know

Before turning attention to how training affects the body's ability to use oxygen, let's examine four terms associated with oxygen consumption. The first term is *respiratory exchange ratio* (RER). Although RER has little practical value outside the laboratory, you should be aware of what it means and how it is used. Without getting too technical, RER is the ratio between oxygen use and carbon dioxide production, calculated by dividing the volume of CO_2 produced each minute by the volume of O_2 used each minute:

$$RER = \frac{\dot{V}CO_2}{\dot{V}O_2}$$

RER is used to estimate how much fat and carbohydrate are oxidized to produce ATP. Your body is always using both carbohydrate and fat to produce ATP, but the ratio of the two fuel sources changes depending on exercise intensity. At rest, when the need for O_2 is low and fat is being oxidized to produce ATP, the RER value is low. During intense exercise, when muscles are oxidizing mostly

Why Does Maximal Heart Rate Decline With Age?

One of the physiological changes that occurs with aging is a decline in maximal heart rate. In fact, maximal heart rate declines roughly 1 beat per minute per year. That simple fact is the basis for the most common equation for estimating maximal heart rate: $HR_{max} = 220 - age$. However, that equation provides only a very rough estimate of HR_{max}. A more accurate equation is $HR_{max} = [208 - (0.7 \times age)]$. Compare the two equations:

Age	220 − age	[208 − (0.7 × age)]
20	200	194
30	190	187
40	180	180
50	170	173
60	160	166
70	150	159
80	140	152

You can see that the differences between the two equations range from 0 to 12 beats per minute (bpm) across this age range. That's not a huge numerical difference. The real difference lies in how accurately the equations predict HR_{max} in large groups of people. With that in mind, the second equation is a more accurate predictor of HR_{max} than the first one. From a practical standpoint, if you are leading a large group of exercisers and you want each person to have a sense of his or her HR_{max}, use [208 − (0.7 × age)] to make those estimates.

You know that a decline in HR_{max} is inevitable for everyone, and it doesn't matter if you're sedentary or highly fit. But *why* does HR_{max} decline? The answer is not known for certain, but it seems to be that with age, the electrical properties of the heart operate more slowly and the heart becomes less sensitive to hormones such as epinephrine (adrenaline). During the aging process, stroke volume (the volume of blood pumped by each beat of the heart) also declines slightly, perhaps by 10% to 20%. Remember that cardiac output is a product of heart rate and stroke volume (CO = HR × SV), so it should be no surprise that cardiac output declines with age. And that's not all. Because cardiac output is a major determinant of $\dot{V}O_{2max}$, $\dot{V}O_{2max}$ also declines with age.

carbohydrate to produce ATP, the RER is higher. You know that 1 gram of fat is the equivalent of 9 Calories, whereas 1 gram of carbohydrate is 4 Calories. The RER value reflects the ratio between fat and carbohydrate oxidation.

Oxygen deficit is another term you need to understand. Figure 3.5 is a graph that shows oxygen uptake during and after intense exercise.

As the graph shows, metabolic rate remains elevated for hours after stopping exercise. This response is referred to as *excess postexercise oxygen consumption*, or EPOC. The term *oxygen debt* describes the same response, but EPOC is the preferred term. There are many reasons why oxygen consumption remains elevated after exercise, especially after strenuous exercise. It takes a few minutes for breathing and heart rate to return to resting levels, body temperature stays high for a while, stress hormones such as epinephrine (adrenaline) and norepinephrine are elevated, and ATP and PCr stores have to be replenished, as do hemoglobin and myoglobin stores of oxygen. For all those reasons and more, oxygen consumption remains above normal resting level for minutes or sometimes hours after a workout. The longer and harder you exercise, the longer the elevation in EPOC.

You now have at least a basic understanding of $\dot{V}O_{2max}$, but you may have also heard of $\dot{V}O_{2peak}$ and wondered about the difference between the two. It's really pretty simple. $\dot{V}O_{2max}$ describes *maximal* oxygen consumption, typically measured during running, when virtually all muscle groups are active and using oxygen. $\dot{V}O_{2peak}$ refers to the highest oxygen consumption measured during a specific exercise. For example, in cycling the legs are very active, but the upper body musculature is less active. As a result, oxygen consumption is lower but may still be at its peak for that activity. This is a bit of scientific hair splitting, but it's helpful to know the difference between the two terms when clients, athletes, coaches, or students ask.

Heart rate increases during exercise because of changes in nerve input to the heart's pacemaker cells. Once exercise is stopped, the nerve input slowly decreases and so does heart rate.

2 Because it takes your body a few minutes to gear up all the systems needed to increase aerobic ATP production, muscles rely on anaerobic ATP production by the phosphocreatine and glycolytic systems, creating an O_2 deficit. This corresponds to the heavy breathing and excess strain you feel right at the beginning of exercise.

3 *Oxygen deficit* refers to how much oxygen would have been used if the aerobic system were able to produce all the ATP from the very second that exercise began.

4 Once your aerobic energy system is up and running, your muscles rely less on the anaerobic systems. You settle in and feel like your body has adapted to the exercise intensity.

1 Whenever you begin any physical activity, your muscles have to suddenly increase ATP production from a very low level at rest to a much higher level during exercise.

5 When you stop a bout of exercise, your oxygen consumption (metabolic rate) remains elevated even though you're no longer producing ATP at a high rate. In fact, oxygen consumption can remain above normal resting values for many hours after exercise.

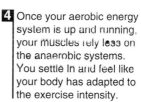
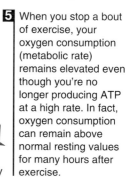

FIGURE 3.5 The oxygen deficit refers to how much oxygen would be needed to cover ATP production at the start of exercise. EPOC is the excess oxygen consumption after exercise has ended.

Adapted, by permission, from W.L. Kenney, J.H. Wilmore, and D.L. Costill, 2015, *Physiology of sport and exercise*, 6th ed. (Champaign, IL: Human Kinetics), 129.

How Does Training Help the Body Use More Oxygen?

Chapter 1 contains a list of many of the adaptations that occur with aerobic (endurance) training. Most of those adaptations are related to increasing the body's capacity to use oxygen. For instance, aerobic training stimulates muscle cells to increase their mitochondrial content as well as the enzymes associated with the Krebs cycle and the electron transport chain. To take full advantage of those adaptations, the body also has to be able to deliver more oxygen to muscle cells. That's accomplished by adaptations in the cardiorespiratory system. Two critical adaptations are an increase in cardiac output and an increase in muscle blood flow. In fact, a greater cardiac output makes the greatest total contribution to increasing $\dot{V}O_{2max}$.

You might recall that cardiac output is determined by heart rate and stroke volume (CO = HR $\times$ SV). Although training does not alter maximum heart rate, training does increase stroke volume (the volume of blood pumped with each beat of the heart). Stroke volume increases with training because the heart's left ventricle becomes a larger and stronger pump, pushing out more blood with each beat. Blood volume (the total amount of blood in the body) also increases with training, enabling the heart to increase its output. Because $\dot{V}O_{2max}$ is determined by cardiac output and the muscles' ability to extract oxygen from the blood, proper aerobic training results in increased $\dot{V}O_{2max}$. If you've studied exercise physiology, you might remember the Fick equation: $\dot{V}O_2 = CO \times a\text{-}\bar{v}O_{2diff}$. In simple terms, this equation states that $\dot{V}O_2$ increases whenever cardiac output and oxygen extraction increase. (The a-$\bar{v}O_{2diff}$ refers to the difference between the oxygen content of blood in arteries and in veins; a larger value means that more oxygen has been extracted and used.)

During an exercise bout, the body must make many adjustments to ensure that all cells receive an adequate supply of blood, oxygen, and nutrients. Because active muscles need more blood, oxygen, and nutrients than less active cells, the body makes the necessary adjustments. Follow the steps shown in figure 3.6 for a summary of the key adjustments that occur in the cardiovascular system.

Blood volume decreases during exercise for three reasons: Some blood plasma is pushed out of the vessels as the result of the increase in blood pressure, some plasma is drawn from the vessels into muscle cells, and some plasma water is lost as sweat. To cope with the decrease in blood volume that occurs during exercise, heart rate increases to help maintain cardiac output.

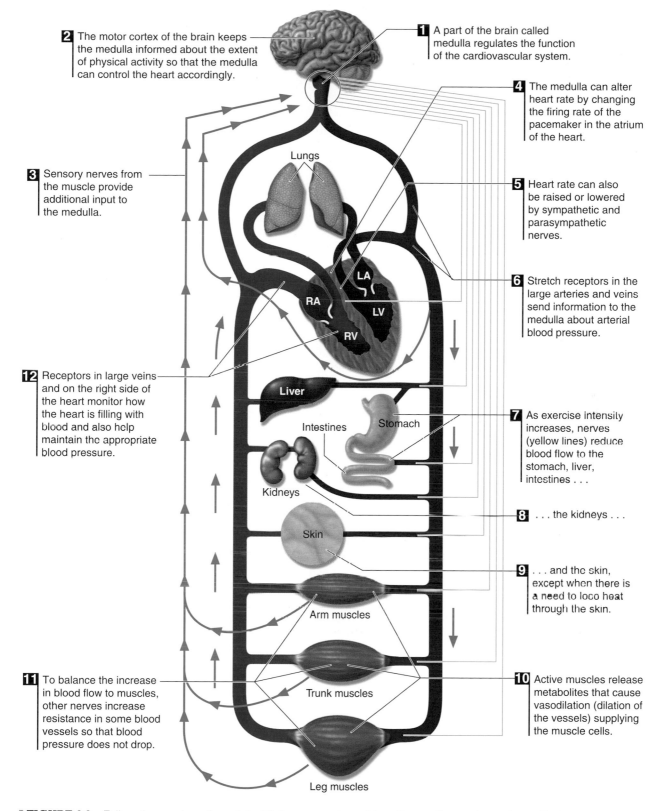

2 The motor cortex of the brain keeps the medulla informed about the extent of physical activity so that the medulla can control the heart accordingly.

1 A part of the brain called medulla regulates the function of the cardiovascular system.

4 The medulla can alter heart rate by changing the firing rate of the pacemaker in the atrium of the heart.

3 Sensory nerves from the muscle provide additional input to the medulla.

5 Heart rate can also be raised or lowered by sympathetic and parasympathetic nerves.

6 Stretch receptors in the large arteries and veins send information to the medulla about arterial blood pressure.

12 Receptors in large veins and on the right side of the heart monitor how the heart is filling with blood and also help maintain the appropriate blood pressure.

7 As exercise intensity increases, nerves (yellow lines) reduce blood flow to the stomach, liver, intestines . . .

8 . . . the kidneys . . .

9 . . . and the skin, except when there is a need to lose heat through the skin.

11 To balance the increase in blood flow to muscles, other nerves increase resistance in some blood vessels so that blood pressure does not drop.

10 Active muscles release metabolites that cause vasodilation (dilation of the vessels) supplying the muscle cells.

Lungs

LA

RA

LV

RV

Liver

Intestines

Stomach

Kidneys

Skin

Arm muscles

Trunk muscles

Leg muscles

FIGURE 3.6 Follow the numbers from 1 to 12 for an overview of how the cardiovascular system adjusts to exercise to ensure that adequate blood, oxygen, and nutrients are delivered to active muscles.

Adapted, by permission, from E.F. Coyle, 1991, "Cardiovascular function during exercise: Neural control factors," *Sports Science Exchange* 4(34): 1-6. Copyright 1991 by Gatorade Sports Science Institute.

One of the many benefits of regular exercise is maintenance of healthy blood pressure. High blood pressure (hypertension) is associated with increased risk of heart attack and stroke, which is why doctors and nurses check the blood pressure of patients during every office visit. The average "normal" blood pressure is 120/80. These numbers are just shorthand to indicate that the blood pressure reading registered 120 mmHg (millimeters of mercury is a unit that depicts pressure) in the large arteries (such as in the upper arm, where the blood pressure cuff is placed) and 80 mmHg between heartbeats, when the heart is at rest. The higher number is referred to as systolic pressure; the lower number is diastolic pressure. During exercise, systolic pressure rises as exercise intensity increases. Diastolic pressure remains the same or may even drop a bit. Improving fitness does not alter resting blood pressure in healthy people but can reduce both systolic and diastolic pressures by 6 to 7 mmHg in people with hypertension.

What Limits Aerobic Endurance Capacity?

If you train smart and hard, why can't you continue to improve your $\dot{V}O_{2max}$? It turns out that the major limit to aerobic capacity has to do with oxygen delivery to active muscles. Muscles of fit endurance athletes have enough mitochondria and oxidative enzymes to handle the oxygen delivered in the bloodstream. In fact, endurance performance is improved when exercisers breathe air enriched with oxygen, showing that muscles are capable of using more oxygen than what is normally delivered to them. The supply of oxygen to muscles limits aerobic capacity. In other words, the upper limits of cardiac output and muscle blood flow establish a top end for aerobic capacity ($\dot{V}O_{2max}$).

Even though being out of breath is always associated with hard exercise, breathing does not limit performance in healthy exercisers. That means that the lungs are capable of supplying as much oxygen as muscles can handle, but the muscles reach their maximal capacity to use the oxygen before the lungs reach their limit to deliver oxygen into the blood.

Improving Aerobic Capacity

If you were to create a training plan to maximize a person's aerobic capacity, what should be the length of the training program? Three months? Six months? Two years? More?

Research indicates that a person's highest attainable $\dot{V}O_{2max}$ can be achieved after roughly 12 to 18 months of proper training. Fortunately, even though $\dot{V}O_{2max}$ may hit a limit, endurance performance can continue to improve because training can increase the lactate threshold, allowing endurance athletes to maintain a faster pace.

The 12- to 18-month time frame to improve $\dot{V}O_{2max}$ is likely true for most people, but as with all physiological adaptations, some people will take considerably more time and others will take less time. This *biological variability* among people is due to a few factors. First, you won't be surprised to learn that heredity plays a major role in response to a training program, accounting for perhaps 50% of capacity to improve $\dot{V}O_{2max}$. As unfair as it may seem, some untrained people with no history of endurance training have high $\dot{V}O_{2max}$ values (e.g., >60 ml/kg/min). Lucky them.

Initial training status also affects how much $\dot{V}O_{2max}$ can increase. For example, a client who is new to fitness training has a greater opportunity to improve his $\dot{V}O_{2max}$ than a client who has been training on and off. Both clients can achieve higher $\dot{V}O_{2max}$ values, but the untrained client will experience a larger relative improvement.

If you are a woman, your $\dot{V}O_{2max}$ value, on average, will be about 10% less than that of a man of similar age and training status. That difference may not mean much when it comes time to race, because it's common for female runners, swimmers, cyclists, and rowers to post faster times than many men. This reality reflects individual variation among men and women and is one more example of why $\dot{V}O_{2max}$ is not a good predictor of endurance performance.

Recall from chapter 1 that some people are high responders to training while others are low responders, and that's certainly true of improvements in $\dot{V}O_{2max}$. Imagine a group of people with similar $\dot{V}O_{2max}$ values who then complete a 12-week endurance training program. Improvements in individual $\dot{V}O_{2max}$ values in response to such a training program may range from 0% to 50%. Imagine how frustrating it must be to train hard and have no improvement in $\dot{V}O_{2max}$!

A benefit of aerobic training is the increased production of red blood cells. But the percentage of blood taken up by red blood cells (known as the hematocrit) actually falls over the first couple of weeks of training because the increase in blood volume is greater than the increase in red blood cells. Hematocrit eventually returns to normal, and performance benefits from both the increase in blood volume and the increase in number of red blood cells.

Oxygen Delivery and Performance Enhancement

Proper training can increase oxygen delivery to active muscles by increasing cardiac output, maximal blood flow, and capillary density in active muscles. Those are the adaptations that enable improvements in endurance performance. But as some athletes have shown, there are other ways to improve oxygen delivery and endurance performance.

Prohibited Techniques

Blood doping is one illegal approach to increasing aerobic capacity. Removing and storing blood from an athlete, waiting a few weeks for the athlete's body to replenish the lost blood, and then infusing the stored blood into the athlete result in increased oxygen delivery and improved performance. Blood doping increases blood volume and hemoglobin content so that more blood and oxygen can be delivered to active muscles. The World Anti-Doping Agency, the U.S. Anti-Doping Agency, and other sport governing bodies consider blood doping as cheating because it is a shortcut to improved performance that is not the result of training.

Another illicit way to increase oxygen delivery is with injections of *erythropoietin* (EPO). EPO is naturally produced by the kidneys to ensure a sufficient number of red blood cells in the bloodstream. EPO promotes the formation of red blood cells by bone marrow. EPO injections result in increased red blood cell production, which means increased hemoglobin and greater oxygen delivery. One risk of using EPO is that too many red blood cells can be produced, increasing the viscosity (thickness) of the blood and creating an enormous strain on the heart. It is thought that dozens of young, healthy competitive cyclists have died of heart attacks related to their use of EPO.

Other Techniques

Some endurance athletes sleep in altitude tents or rooms with a reduced amount of oxygen in the air (lower partial pressure of oxygen, to be precise) to stimulate natural EPO production and increase the red blood cell content of their blood. Those techniques for increasing red blood cell mass are not illegal. Competitive swimmers often engage in *hypoxic training* by reducing their breathing frequency or holding their breath during repeat swims. Elite distance runners often spend time at altitude to try to benefit from exposure to the hypoxic (lower-than-normal oxygen content) environment, a topic covered in more detail in chapter 10. The intent of hypoxic training is to induce physiological and metabolic changes that promote greater adaptations. Research shows that living at high altitude (>1,650 ft, or >500 m, above sea level) and training at low altitude (<1,650 ft) improve $\dot{V}O_{2max}$ and endurance performance in part because of an increase in red blood cell production.

For athletes interested in improving muscle strength, a variation of hypoxic training is *blood flow restriction*, in which the blood flow to arms or legs is reduced during strength training to create a greater training stress. It appears that blood flow restriction can also promote positive changes that result in improved strength and muscle mass.

For most people, it does not make sense to live at altitude, sleep in altitude tents, or restrict blood flow during strength training. A simpler solution for those looking for improved performance is to alter the intensity, duration, and frequency of training to create a progressively increasing training stress.

Breathing oxygen-enriched air from a tank improves endurance performance by increasing oxygen delivery to active muscles. Even though red blood cell hemoglobin is almost always completely saturated with oxygen (about 98% of the hemoglobin in blood is saturated with oxygen), breathing 100% oxygen will increase the amount of oxygen in blood by about 10%, enough to improve endurance performance. For mountain climbers at high altitude, it makes sense to carry an oxygen tank to help ensure improved performance and safety. That's not true for athletes in any other sport except scuba diving.

What about breathing 100% oxygen during recovery, as American football players are often seen doing on the sidelines? Sport scientists have not been able to find a physiological benefit to breathing oxygen during recovery. In other words, breathing oxygen during recovery does not improve performance in a subsequent bout of exercise. This continuing practice is a good example of the *placebo effect*—when psychological expectations trump physiological benefits. For that reason alone, oxygen tanks are unlikely to disappear from football sidelines.

Eating more vegetables might actually be an effective way to improve endurance performance. Vegetables such as celery, carrots, beets, and rhubarb contain nitrates, a simple combination of one nitrogen atom linked to three oxygen atoms. In the body, nitrates are converted into the biologically active compound nitric oxide (1 nitrogen and 1 oxygen). Research shows that increasing nitric oxide in muscle cells helps reduce the oxygen cost of exercise and improve endurance performance. In other words, less oxygen is used during exercise even though the exercise intensity is unchanged. From a health standpoint, nitrate ingestion is associated with lower blood pressure, a real plus for those who struggle with hypertension.

CHAPTER FOUR

Fatigue: What Is It Good For?

Fatigue has many causes but also many benefits in maximizing adaptations to exercise training.

No one likes to become fatigued, even though it's a natural consequence of tough exercise. Fatigue saps physical capacity, drains mental focus, and exhausts the desire to maintain the pace of exercise. Fatigue is often equated with failure, especially when fatigue occurs during competition. After all, one of the most important benefits of training is to delay the onset of fatigue for as long as possible. Whether you're sprinting 100 meters or pacing yourself through a marathon, fatigue is what slows you down. Fatigue—physical or mental—simply refers to the inability to maintain *a task*.

You know from personal experience that fatigue comes in various forms. The mental fatigue you encounter after a long day in the office feels different from the fatigue of a long day of physical labor. The intense fatigue that accompanies a 400-meter track race is not at all like the fatigue resulting from a marathon run. Yet, in both cases fatigue limits the ability to maintain a fast pace. The stark difference in how you sense fatigue is an indication that fatigue has various causes that are related to the intensity and duration of exercise.

Jacob Ammentorp Lund/iStock

What Causes Fatigue?

Table 4.1 is a list of the mechanisms by which fatigue can occur. For example, fatigue can occur as a result of peripheral reasons that limit the ability of muscle cells to produce ATP molecules at a rate required to maintain the desired intensity of exercise. Fatigue can also occur as the result of central limitations, or the inability of the brain and nervous system to maintain the requirements of continued exercise. Central fatigue can take the form of losing the desire or motivation to continue exercise or a decline in some aspect of the motor skills associated with continued exercise. In other words, you lose focus, become uncoordinated, and either slow down or stop. Some scientists suggest that central fatigue helps protect highly motivated athletes from pushing themselves too far, even beyond the point when peripheral fatigue would cause most people to stop.

To help you understand how fatigue occurs and how training, nutrition, and hydration can help delay the onset of fatigue and improve performance, take a brief look at each cause of fatigue and its underlying mechanisms.

During brief, all-out efforts, muscle cells are capable of increasing the rate of ATP production 1,000 times that of rest. Any factor that reduces the rate of ATP production required to sustain a certain exercise intensity will result in fatigue.

TABLE 4.1 **Possible Causes of Fatigue During Exercise**

Cause	What it means	How it limits exercise
PCr depletion	Cells run short of the phosphocreatine used to quickly generate ATP	Reduces the capacity for high-intensity contractions
ATP depletion	When ATP cannot be produced at the needed rate, overall levels in muscle cells drop	Reduces the capacity for high-intensity contractions
Glycogen depletion	Glycogen deposits, the storage form of glucose in muscles and liver, fall to low levels	Less glucose is available for use as fuel, reducing the rate at which muscle cells can produce ATP
Hypoglycemia	Low blood sugar	Reduces the uptake and use of glucose by brain, nerves, and muscle cells, making exercise feel more difficult
Hypovolemia	Low blood volume, often due to dehydration	Reduces cardiac output, the ability of the heart to supply blood to working muscles
Hyperthermia	High body temperature	Makes exercise feel more difficult and reduces the brain's desire to continue exercise
Metabolic acidosis	An accumulation of lactate molecules and hydrogen ions in blood and muscles	Reduces the ability of muscle cells to contract. Increases breathing rate.
Disrupted neural transmission	Impaired nerve function	Alters signals to and from muscle, negatively affecting coordination and strength
Disrupted brain activity	Impaired brain function	Reduces the desire to continue exercise and the muscular coordination required to maintain exercise

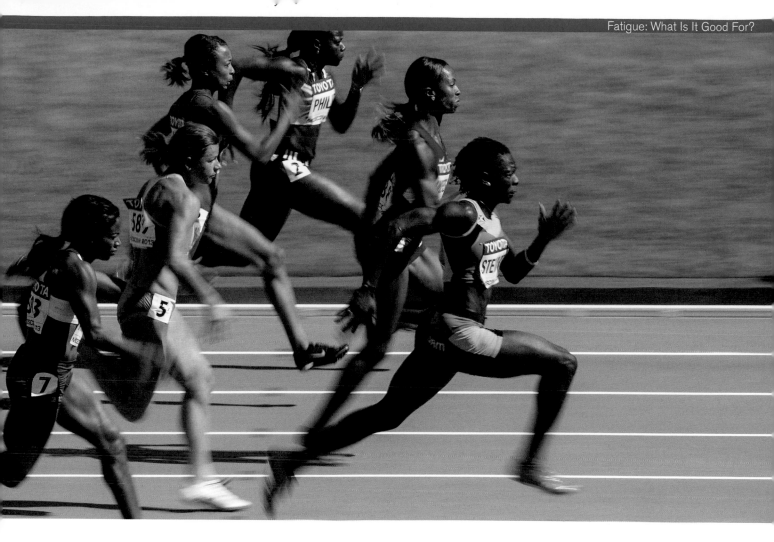

Phosphocreatine and ATP Depletion

These two factors are discussed together because they are so closely related during high-intensity efforts. In figure 4.1 you'll see that at the start of all-out exercise, PCr is quickly broken down to form the ATP needed for rapid muscle contraction. Some of the ATP molecules stored inside muscle cells are also used for muscle contraction. That combination

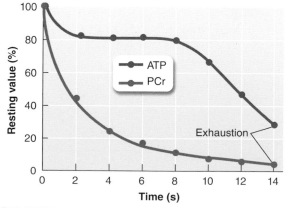

FIGURE 4.1 PCr and ATP levels fall quickly during all-out exercise.

of PCr and ATP is enough to maintain all-out exercise for only a few seconds, but that's long enough to allow for glycolysis to ramp up ATP production. As you can imagine, all-out exercise quickly reduces the supply of PCr in active muscle cells. ATP supplies also drop quickly but never fall as much as PCr levels because ATP is continuously produced by other pathways. Once PCr and ATP supplies fall sufficiently, the pace of exercise begins to slow because the rate of overall ATP production has slowed. That's why even the world's elite sprinters can maintain top speed for only about 4 seconds before they begin to slow.

It would be a waste of money to buy ATP and PCr supplements because both molecules are broken down during digestion. However, consuming creatine supplements has been shown to increase muscle PCr stores, at least in those study participants whose muscle creatine stores are not already at maximum. Creatine supplementation has also been shown to increase performance in repeated bursts of high-intensity exercise. This change may enhance the response to intense interval training by allowing more intense training sessions.

63

Glycogen Depletion

Whenever muscles contract, the large glycogen molecules inside the active muscle cells are continuously broken down to supply most of the glucose molecules that enter glycolysis to begin the production of ATP. Glycogen is a critical fuel for muscles; when glycogen stores fall to low levels, exercise feels much more difficult and performance is impaired. Figure 4.2 shows that as glycogen levels fell in the gastrocnemius muscle during treadmill running, the participant rated the exercise to be more and more difficult, even though his running speed remained unchanged.

Muscle glycogen can definitely be a limiting factor during endurance exercise, but keep in mind that high-intensity exercise also relies on muscle glycogen. In fact, the rate at which muscle glycogen is broken down during sprinting can be 40 times faster than the rate during walking. You might have also noticed in figure 4.2 that during the first hour of treadmill running, muscle glycogen stores fell faster than after the first hour. Muscles are happy to break down glycogen to produce ATP and do so whenever glycogen levels are high. Later in exercise, as glycogen levels drop, muscles rely more on the oxidation of fatty acids to produce ATP, causing reduced speed or, as in the case of the person in figure 4.2, continued exercise at the same pace as the discomfort in doing so grows. In this example, you might say that the person "hit the wall" after about 1.5 hours of treadmill running, the point at which low muscle glycogen was associated with a large increase in perceived exertion.

The intensity of exercise determines how rapidly muscle glycogen is broken down; the more intense the exercise, the faster the rate of glycogen depletion. From a practical standpoint, anyone who trains hard should consume a diet

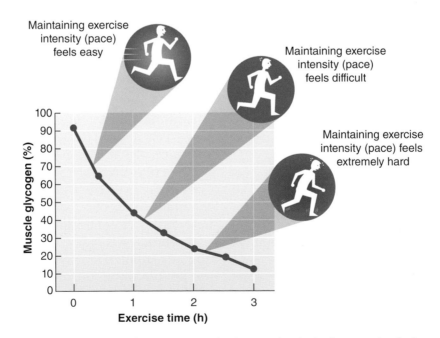

FIGURE 4.2 During prolonged exercise, muscle glycogen levels decline, exercise feels much more difficult, and pace slows.

Adapted, by permission, from D.L. Costill, 1986, *Inside running: Basics of sports physiology* (Indianapolis: Benchmark Press). Copyright 1986 Cooper Publishing Group, Carmel, IN.

high in carbohydrate to replace the muscle glycogen used during training. High-carbohydrate diets are not just for endurance athletes.

Also remember that the type of exercise affects how muscle glycogen is used. For example, sprinters use more glycogen from their type II fibers, while endurance athletes use more glycogen from their type I fibers. Other factors influence how active muscle cells use their muscle glycogen. For example, glycogen is depleted at various rates depending on which muscles are most stressed by a particular exercise. In figure 4.3 you'll see that running on the level, uphill, or downhill determines which muscles use the most glycogen.

If muscle glycogen is so important to performance, what is the best way to protect glycogen stores? For example, by consuming carbohydrate during exercise, can you slow the use of muscle glycogen? Unfortunately, the answer to that question seems to be no. Consuming a sports drink, energy bar, or carbohydrate gel can certainly improve exercise performance by helping maintain a high rate of overall carbohydrate oxidation, but muscle glycogen use seems to be unaffected.

Consuming carbohydrate during exercise helps maintain blood glucose levels, preventing a drop in blood glucose, or *hypoglycemia*. During both rest and exercise, the liver has the job of adding glucose molecules to the bloodstream to maintain a normal blood sugar (glucose) level. But the liver has a limited supply of its own glycogen; when those stores are depleted, hypoglycemia occurs unless you're able to consume carbohydrate. One of the many reasons to recommend that athletes consume carbohydrate before beginning a morning workout is to help replenish the liver glycogen levels that dropped during sleep.

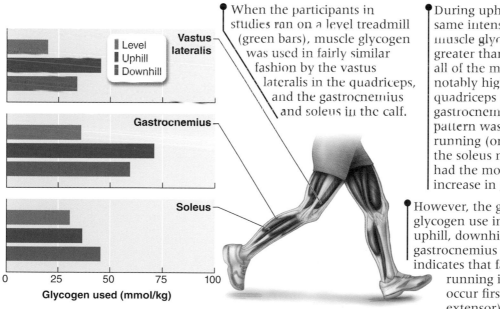

When the participants in studies ran on a level treadmill (green bars), muscle glycogen was used in fairly similar fashion by the vastus lateralis in the quadriceps, and the gastrocnemius and soleus in the calf.

During uphill running at the same intensity (blue bars), muscle glycogen use was greater than in level running in all of the muscle groups but notably higher in the quadriceps and the gastrocnemius. A different pattern was seen with downhill running (orange bars), where the soleus muscle in the calf had the most pronounced increase in glycogen use.

However, the greatest muscle glycogen use in all cases (level, uphill, downhill) occurred in the gastrocnemius (calf) muscle. This indicates that fatigue during running is most likely to occur first in the calf (ankle extensor) muscles.

FIGURE 4.3 Muscle glycogen use in three sets of leg muscles during treadmill running on the level, uphill, and downhill.

Adapted, by permission, from W.L. Kenney, J.H. Wilmore, and D.L. Costill, 2015, *Physiology of sport and exercise*, 6th ed. (Champaign, IL: Human Kinetics), 136.

Hypoglycemia

As noted previously, when the liver runs low on glycogen, blood sugar level falls and hypoglycemia results. Symptoms include mental and physical fatigue, shakiness and weakness, and hunger. Understandably, consuming carbohydrate during exercise helps maintain blood sugar and spares liver glycogen. When exhausted people who have exercised for hours without consuming carbohydrate are fed a few hundred Calories of simple sugar, they are able to continue exercise. The reason that consuming carbohydrate has such a major impact on exercise performance is that maintaining blood glucose concentration not only ensures that active muscles have a steady supply of glucose for ATP production, but it also does the same for the brain and nerves. The central nervous system is an obligatory user of glucose for ATP production. In other words, under normal circumstances, glucose is the only fuel used by the brain and nerves. That's why hypoglycemia can cause fatigue and irritability.

Effects of Dehydration

Increased

Incidence of GI discomfort

Plasma osmolality

Blood viscosity

Heart rate

Resting core temperature

Skin temperature

Brain temperature

Core temperature at which sweating begins

Core temperature at which skin blood flow increases

Core temperature at a given $\dot{V}O_2$

Carbohydrate oxidation

Glycogen breakdown in muscle and liver

Thermal discomfort

Decreased

Blood plasma volume

Blood flow to internal organs

Central blood volume

Central venous pressure

Cardiac filling pressure

Stroke volume

Cardiac output

Skin blood flow at a given core temperature

Maximal skin blood flow

Muscle blood flow

Sweat rate at a given core temperature

Maximal sweat rate

Glycogen synthesis in muscle and liver

Physical and mental performance

Dehydration

Hypovolemia is the medical term for lower-than-normal blood volume, one of the main effects of dehydration. Most people are more familiar with the term *dehydration*, so that's the term used in this text from now on.

Sweating is a real challenge to fluid regulation because the water molecules in sweat come from the bloodstream (*vascular fluid*), from fluid that bathes the cells (*interstitial fluid*), and from fluid inside the cells (*intracellular fluid*). If you work up a big sweat, it's easy to lose water from the body a lot faster than you're able to drink it. As a result, you become dehydrated.

Even slight dehydration (e.g., a loss of 1% of body weight, just 2 pounds for a 200-pound person) results in measurable physiological changes. As dehydration worsens, so do the effects on physiology and performance, especially in warm environments. Dehydration impairs a variety of physiological functions, making it difficult and uncomfortable to maintain exercise intensity.

It is important to avoid dehydration, which is easily accomplished in most cases by drinking during exercise. Staying well hydrated during physical activity helps you get the most out of your body, makes exercise more comfortable, and decreases the risk of heat illness. But how much should you drink during exercise? That question has no single answer because everyone sweats at a different rate. Some people are light sweaters (<1 L/hr) and sweat only enough to moisten the skin. Most people are average sweaters (1-2 L/hr) and some people are heavy sweaters (>2 L/hr). Figure 4.4 is a simple depiction of how widely sweating rates can vary among people.

Regardless of sweating rate, the goal is to drink enough during exercise to minimize loss of body weight. That's why weighing before and after exercise is helpful for anyone who works up a sweat on a regular basis. Loss of greater than 2 percent of body weight indicates dehydration and the need to increase fluid intake during future training sessions. A gain in body weight indicates that too much fluid has been consumed.

Putting aside scientific details, here is the practical message about hydration: It's always better to be well hydrated than dehydrated. That's true for overall health and particularly true for ability to perform optimally, both physically and mentally.

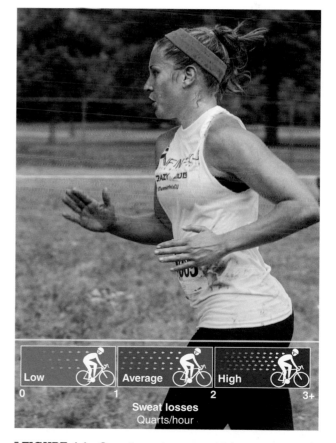

FIGURE 4.4 Sweating rates vary widely among people depending on genetic predisposition to sweating, fitness, ambient temperature, exercise intensity, and other factors.

Hyperthermia

One of the unavoidable effects of dehydration is an increase in core body temperature. But *hyperthermia* can also occur in well-hydrated people either as a result of exercise in a warm environment or simply as the result of exposure to a hot environment, such as a sauna.

Body temperature naturally rises during physical activity because heat is a by-product of muscle contraction. Too much of a rise in body temperature (often referred to as *core temperature*) impairs performance and increases the risk of heat illnesses such as *heat exhaustion* and *heatstroke*. A quick look at figure 4.5 confirms that heat impairs exercise performance. Heat limits the ability to exercise because core temperature rises, muscle glycogen is broken down faster, blood is redirected to the skin to aid in heat loss, sweating rate is greater, the risk of dehydration increases, and the motivation to continue exercise lessens.

Research studies have shown that precooling muscles improves performance and preheating muscles impairs performance. That's one reason why athletes warming up for a training session or competition on a hot day should do just that—warm up, not heat up.

Hyperthermia is bad news for performance because a hot body—and a hot brain—don't function optimally. In fact, high body temperature limits capacity and desire for exercise by negatively affecting the function of the cardiovascular system, muscles, and brain. As you heat up, the heart has to pump more blood to the skin to aid in heat loss, reducing blood flow to muscles, especially when you allow yourself to dehydrate. Heat also saps the brain's desire to continue exercise, causing most people to slow or stop as a way to reduce heat production and prevent heat illness. Staying well hydrated and using strategies to reduce heat gain during exercise—such as taking advantage of the wind and shade, removing some clothing, and reducing exercise intensity—can prevent hyperthermia and its negative impact on performance.

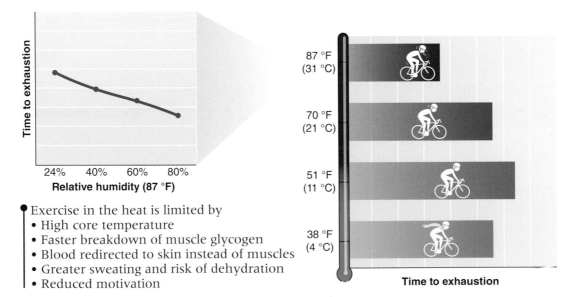

Exercise in the heat is limited by
- High core temperature
- Faster breakdown of muscle glycogen
- Blood redirected to skin instead of muscles
- Greater sweating and risk of dehydration
- Reduced motivation

FIGURE 4.5 Heat impairs exercise performance. Studies show that at higher temperature and humidity, run times to exhaustion are reduced.

Part a data from S.D.R. Galloway and R.J. Maughan, 1997, "Effects of ambient temperature on the capacity to perform prolonged cycle exercise in man," *Medicine and Science in Sports and Exercise* 29: 1240-1249; part b data from R.J. Maughan et al., 2012, "Influence of relative humidity on prolonged exercise capacity in a warm environment," *European Journal of Applied Physiology* 112: 2313-2321.

Metabolic Acidosis

You know from experience that you can't maintain intense exercise very long before doing so becomes uncomfortable and you are forced to slow down. That type of fatigue is often blamed on the buildup of lactic acid, which is partially true. Intense exercise does generate a lot of lactic acid as a by-product of the production of ATP through anaerobic glycolysis. In fact, when lactic acid rapidly accumulates inside muscle cells, it *dissociates* (breaks apart) into a lactate molecule and a hydrogen ion (H^+). The lactate molecule can be converted back into a pyruvate molecule and enter the citric acid cycle to help produce more ATP. Or the lactate molecule can diffuse out of the muscle cell into the bloodstream, where it can be picked up by other tissues, converted to pyruvate, and used for ATP production.

The H^+ ion is the real troublemaker. As H^+ ions accumulate inside muscle cells, the pH of the cell rapidly drops. In other words, the cell becomes more acidic and that reduces the cell's ability to produce ATP from glycolysis. Fortunately, muscle cells contain buffer systems that prevent pH from dropping so low that it damages the cell (figure 4.6). But the slight acidification that does occur limits the ability to continue intense exercise because it limits ATP production and muscle contraction.

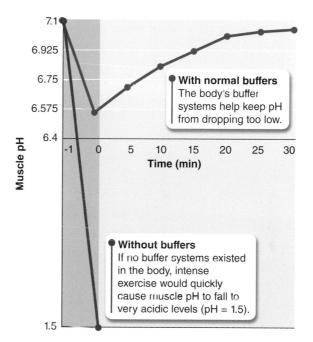

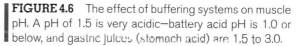

FIGURE 4.6 The effect of buffering systems on muscle pH. A pH of 1.5 is very acidic—battery acid pH is 1.0 or below, and gastric juices (stomach acid) are 1.5 to 3.0.

Precooling Aids Performance

Getting too hot impairs performance, and getting too cold does likewise. But keeping core temperature from climbing too high too fast can benefit performance. Staying well hydrated during exercise in the heat is one way to accomplish that, and becoming acclimated to the heat is another. So is precooling the body before intense exercise. Core temperature can be lowered slightly by consuming ice-slushy drinks, wearing a cooling vest, or sitting in cold water or a cold room. Beginning intense exercise cooler than normal increases the time it takes for core temperature to climb to levels that can impair performance.

Research shows that precooling can improve performance, especially with prolonged exercise in warm environments, when high body temperature can adversely affect the mental desire and physical capacity to continue intense exercise. It is clear that precooling strategies have to be adjusted to the conditions of training and competition that vary greatly among sports, but precooling is a strategy worth considering for anyone—athlete, soldier, or worker—who is physically active in hot environments.

One of the ways that a drop

in muscle cell pH impairs performance is thought to be interference with how calcium ions (Ca^{2+}) function in the contractile process (figure 4.7). Recall from chapter 1 that muscle contraction depends on the release of Ca^{2+} ions from the sarcoplasmic reticulum, followed by the equally rapid uptake of Ca^{2+} ions back into the sarcoplasmic reticulum.

A few studies have reported that people can increase their capacity for intense exercise by consuming solutions containing sodium bicarbonate or sodium citrate. Both bicarbonate and citrate act as buffers to counteract the accumulation of H^+ ions that slow glycolysis and interfere with muscle contractions. Most studies show no effect.

Lactic acid itself does not cause fatigue, but the hydrogen ions produced along with lactic acid cause muscle cells to become acidic, interfering with energy production and muscle contraction.

FIGURE 4.7 Anything that interferes with how Ca^{2+} ions move in and out of the sarcoplasmic reticulum and interact with troponin will cause a reduction in muscle force production—fatigue.

Normal process

The job of Ca^{2+} ions is to bind to troponin, causing tropomyosin strands to move just enough to uncover the active sites on the actin filaments to which myosin heads can bind and cause contraction.

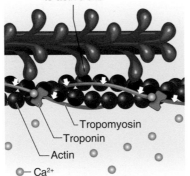

Myosin head bound to active site

Tropomyosin
Troponin
Actin
Ca^{2+}

Interference of hydrogen ions

The accumulation of H+ ions interferes with the function of Ca2+ ions, which causes a decrease in contractile force and fatigue (the inability to maintain a task).

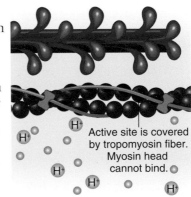

Active site is covered by tropomyosin fiber. Myosin head cannot bind.

H+ H+ H+ H+

Disrupted Neural Transmission

The brain, spine, and neuromuscular junction (point where motor nerves connect to muscle) are all locations where various factors might contribute to fatigue, as depicted in figure 4.8.

The brain is the control center for all voluntary human movements, and this *central drive* to continue exercise can be influenced to alter fatigue. The current thinking is that the brain reduces the drive (desire) to exercise as a way to protect the body from injury or worse. Those protective mechanisms are usually effective but can be overridden by drugs such as amphetamines and by mental distractions. For example, shouting, music, and even verbal encouragement can temporarily increase the strength of muscle contractions, even in muscles that have been fatigued by prior exercise. It's also possible that a highly motivated athlete can push so hard that life is threatened by hyperthermia. Although the brain is programmed to slow run pace during exercise in hot weather where continuing a fast pace could result in heatstroke and death, some athletes have ignored those symptoms with tragic consequences.

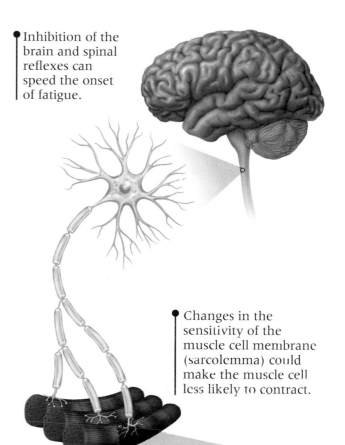

● Inhibition of the brain and spinal reflexes can speed the onset of fatigue.

● Changes in the sensitivity of the muscle cell membrane (sarcolemma) could make the muscle cell less likely to contract.

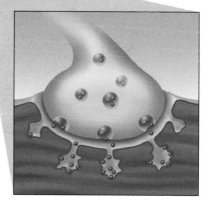

● Reduced release of calcium ions in response to a nervous impulse could cause fatigue.

● Slower release of acetylcholine molecules at the synapse between the motor neuron and the muscle could cause fatigue.

● After it is released and signals a muscle to contract, acetylcholine is broken down by specialized enzymes. Changes in the activity of these enzymes could influence fatigue.

FIGURE 4.8 Changes in the normal operations of the brain, spinal reflexes, and neuromuscular junction can contribute to fatigue.

What's the Difference Between Fatigue and Overtraining?

Fatigue is the inability to continue a task. That could be the inability to continue to curl a dumbbell; the inability to maintain a desired pace on the track, in the pool, or on the bike; or the inability to react quickly to a stimulus. A hallmark of fatigue is that it's temporary. Within a few minutes or a few hours, depending on the exercise task, the ability to perform the task returns. In that regard, fatigue is reversible, and that reversibility makes fatigue very different from overtraining.

What Is Overtraining?

Overtraining refers to physiological maladaptations and performance decrements that can last for days or weeks. Figure 4.9 shows how the normal progression for improved fitness can plateau and then either continue to improve or take a precipitous decline (overtraining).

Motivated athletes and clients are often at risk of overtraining because they tend to ignore symptoms of overtraining in their quest for greater fitness and better performance. Overtraining is a risk not just for endurance athletes. Many sports and types of fitness training, martial arts, strength training, and other physical endeavors require rigorous workouts, often more than once each day, making anyone who trains on a regular basis susceptible to overtraining.

FIGURE 4.9 Overtraining is characterized by physiological maladaptations and performance decrements that occur when the body fails to adapt to the training stimulus.

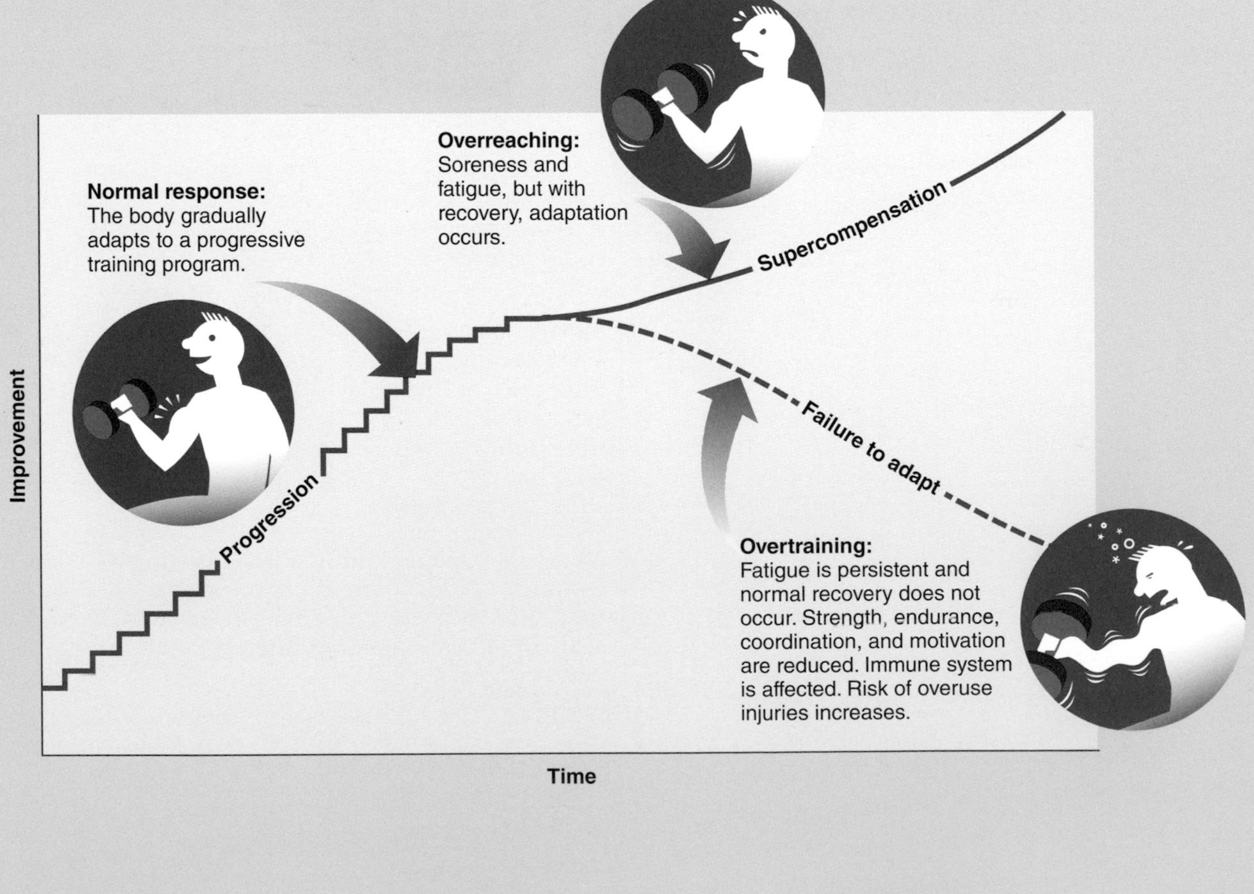

Normal response: The body gradually adapts to a progressive training program.

Overreaching: Soreness and fatigue, but with recovery, adaptation occurs.

Supercompensation

Failure to adapt

Progression

Overtraining: Fatigue is persistent and normal recovery does not occur. Strength, endurance, coordination, and motivation are reduced. Immune system is affected. Risk of overuse injuries increases.

Improvement

Time

What Causes Overtraining?

Excessive training stresses the body beyond its capacity to adapt. But many other stressors raise the risk of overtraining. The emotional demands of balancing training with work or school, the anxiety associated with competition, fear of failure, and the stress of meeting the expectations of coaches and parents all add to the risk of overtraining. Everyone has a unique capacity to deal with physical and emotional stress, so it's no surprise that some athletes will thrive while others fall prey to overtraining, even when they all are exposed to the same amount and type of training. That diversity in response makes it difficult to predict who is susceptible to overtraining. A coach and an athlete often don't realize that the athlete has pushed too hard for too long until it is too late. Scientists have yet to discover a reliable marker that can be used to predict overtraining, but monitoring exercise heart rate seems to be the best approach at this time. Figure 4.10 shows how exercise heart rate during a standardized exercise task fell as a result of training. That decline in exercise heart rate is exactly what is to be expected as a result of a well-designed training program. In this example, when the athlete became overtrained (OT), his exercise heart rate was 15 to 20 bpm *higher* than normal, an indication that his body was struggling to adapt to the stress of training.

You might have heard the term *overreaching* used to describe an important characteristic of training program design. It's important to remember that overreaching is different from overtraining. Coaches and personal trainers realize that the greatest gains in strength and fitness come from training programs that require athletes and clients to regularly push themselves to fatigue (overload). Done correctly, this type of training results in large gains in fitness. Done incorrectly, too much overload leads to overtraining. An important part of the art of coaching—a skill that requires years to develop—is knowing when and how hard to push athletes and when to back off and allow them to rest.

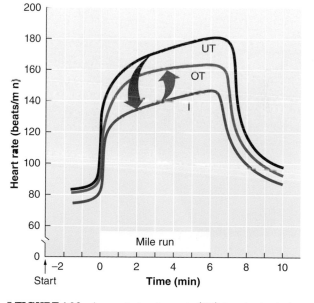

FIGURE 4.10 In overtrained people (OT), heart rate during exercise is higher than normal (T). UT is the heart rate response when the same person is untrained.

Reprinted, by permission, from W.L. Kenney, J.H. Wilmore, and D.L. Costill, 2015, *Physiology of sport and exercise*, 6th ed. (Champaign, IL: Human Kinetics), 358.

© Martin Dimitrow/iStock

Common Symptoms of Overtraining

- Exercise not enjoyable
- Reduced capacity for training (early fatigue)
- Loss of motivation and vigor
- Feelings of depression
- Reduced strength
- Reduced coordination

- Loss of appetite
- Weight loss
- Sleep disturbances
- Irritability
- Inability to focus
- Resting heart rate increased or decreased

- Blood pressure increased or decreased
- Frequent colds
- Chronic muscle soreness
- Irregular menstrual cycles
- Frequent overuse injuries

What Role Does Fatigue Play in Adaptations to Training?

Legendary football coach Vince Lombardi was quoted as saying, "Fatigue makes cowards of us all." That may be true in some cases, but it is also true that fatigue can make better athletes of us all. It is obvious that the human body is well equipped to adapt to the stress of physical training. It should also be obvious that the extent of those adaptations is directly related to the extent of the physical stress. For example, if someone new to exercise begins a strength training program, the total extent of strength gains will depend on the total extent of the training stress. In other words, if the person trains three days each week for six months and lifts progressively heavier weights over that time, that person's strength gains will be greater than that of someone who trains just once each week and does not have much of an increase in training resistance. The overall stress of training is vastly different, so it is no surprise that the overall extent of adaptations will be different.

An obvious index of overall stress is fatigue. Not the kind of all-day, persistent fatigue that is associated with overtraining, but periodic fatigue within training sessions. And not every training session, but at least two times each week for someone training six days per week. Each time you fatigue—whether it's an individual muscle group during strength training or the entire body during endurance training—muscle cells are exposed to hundreds of intracellular signals that result in increased protein production over the next days. Those proteins can be the contractile proteins required for increasing strength and mass, the mitochondrial proteins needed for greater endurance, or the structural proteins used to make muscles and connective tissue more resistant to injury.

Fatigue during exercise maximizes adaptive responses because periodic fatigue maximizes the intracellular signals required to promote those responses. Fatigue that occurs too often sets the stage for overtraining. Adaptations take time, which is why successful coaches understand that they cannot push their athletes hard each day; reducing training stress for a day or two after an intense workout allows time for adaptations (and repair) to occur, enabling athletes to gradually and progressively increase the training stress. Ample rest, sleep, hydration, and nutrition are also required for optimal adaptations.

CHAPTER FIVE

Principles of Designing Training Programs

Strength, power, endurance, agility, and flexibility can all be improved by training programs based on tried-and-true scientific principles.

How hard, how long, and how often should people exercise to achieve their fitness goals? Common sense and science indicate that there is not one simple answer to that question because so many other factors have to be considered in the design of effective training programs. What are the person's goals and expectations? Are those goals related to improved sport performance or other objectives such as weight loss, improved cardiovascular health, or increased muscle mass? When are those goals to be achieved? In two months? Six months? A year? How much time each week can the person devote to training? How old is the person? How experienced? The answers to these and other questions are fundamental to the design of a training program because they determine the expectations and limitations around which a training program is built.

Training programs that are too difficult expose athletes and personal training clients to injury and overtraining syndrome. If the stress of training is not difficult enough, optimal adaptations do not occur and goals are not achieved. Training programs that are too rigid don't allow for innate differences among people to be taken into consideration. The balance between the right amount of exercise needed to optimize adaptations and too much or too little exercise varies widely among people.

What Are the Basics of Program Design?

No matter the goal of the training program—speed, endurance, agility, strength, power, muscle mass, weight loss—you must consider five principles: individuality, specificity, reversibility, progressive overload, and variation. These five scientific principles form the framework for the design of successful training programs.

Five Principles of Program Design

- Individuality. Some people adapt quickly, others slowly, to the same training.
- Specificity. Adaptations are specific to the mode and intensity of training.
- Reversibility. Adaptations to training can be easily lost.
- Progressive overload. A gradual increase in training load prompts improvement.
- Variation. Varying mode, duration, intensity, and frequency maximizes adaptations and reduces the risk of overtraining.

Individuality

The principle of individuality reflects innate differences in the ability to adapt to the stress of exercise. As illustrated in figure 5.1, some people adapt quickly, others slowly, to the same training. In other words, the same training stimulus provokes different amounts and rates of adaptation in different people. As noted in chapter 1, the differences in the adaptive response are largely genetic—some people adapt quickly (high responders), others slowly (low responders). Genetics determines the starting point and the ending point. When designing each program for each client, trainers need to take unique individual characteristics into account and provide the opportunity to maximize adaptive potential through the thoughtful manipulation of exercise intensity, duration, frequency, mode, rest, nutrition, and hydration.

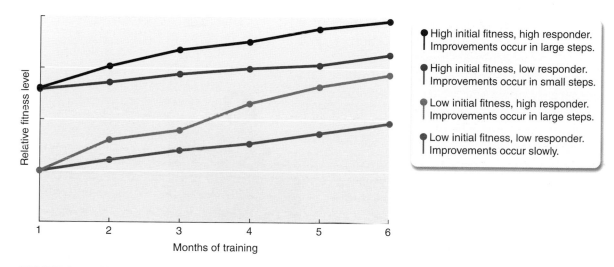

FIGURE 5.1 Both initial fitness and the response to training are affected by genetics and vary among people. Those who design effective training programs take into consideration the fact that people begin training at unique fitness levels and their progress can vary widely depending on their individual capacities to adapt to training.

High-Intensity Interval Training

For untrained and recreationally active individuals, high-intensity interval training (HIIT) can be an effective alternative to traditional endurance training. This is particularly true for people who have limited time to train or are not psychologically prepared for the demands of endurance training. Research has shown that as few as six sessions of HIIT over two weeks—a total of roughly 15 minutes of intense stationary cycling—is enough stimulus to improve exercise capacity and other markers of enhanced endurance. HIIT is typically conducted as repeated short, intense bursts of activity separated by rests of low-intensity activity, so the total time devoted to training over the two-week experiment was only about 2.5 hours. Experts suggest that endurance athletes can optimize training benefits by performing 10% to 15% of their total training as HIIT and conduct the majority of the remaining training at low intensities. HIIT improves maximal oxygen consumption and markers of cardiovascular health with a minimum commitment of time but a maximum commitment of effort.

Reference: Gibala, M.J., & Jones, A.M. (2013). Physiological and performance adaptations to high-intensity interval training. *Nestle Nutrition Institute Workshop Series*, 76:51-60.

Specificity

The principle of specificity holds that most training should reflect the specific demands of the sport or activity. Adaptations are specific to the mode and intensity of training.

Common sense dictates that adaptations in muscles and other tissues will be specific to the stress imposed on them. The adaptations that underlie increased strength and mass are best promoted by resistance training programs that stimulate the production of muscle contractile and structural proteins. For improving endurance capacity, training has to stimulate the production of mitochondrial proteins and adaptation of cardiac tissue to meet the demands of prolonged exercise. Chapter 8 looks at research that shows that high-intensity, short-duration (HIIT) training can increase anaerobic as well as aerobic power and capacity, results that lead to a slightly different interpretation of the principle of specificity. When it comes to specific activities or sports, the principle of specificity holds true: To improve performance in an activity, you should train primarily with that mode of exercise. For example, although competitive swimmers often lift weights, run, cycle, and include plyometrics and other fitness activities in their training, the majority of their training time is in the pool.

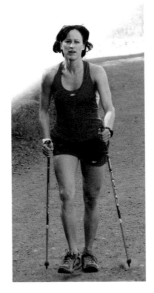

Adaptations to resistance training include increased recruitment of motor units, more contractile filaments, and greater muscle mass (depending in part on the type of resistance training). Additional adaptations are listed in chapter 5.

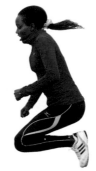

Endurance training results in greater cardiac output, increased $\dot{V}O_{2max}$, and a higher anaerobic threshold, among many other adaptations covered in chapter 9.

Eccentric training can be an important element of training specificity in many sports. Not only does eccentric training help increase muscle mass and strength, but it can also improve the muscles' ability to function as shock absorbers to help prevent landing-related injuries and cope with high external loads in sports such as skiing, ice hockey, and football.

The body adapts to plyometric training with improved neuromuscular coordination, along with increased speed and power, as detailed in chapter 8.

There are occasions when sport-specific training should take an initial back seat to more general training. People who are just beginning a training program—such as adults who want to participate in triathlons but have no experience in the sport—should begin with general training that creates a base fitness level on which sport-specific training can be added. This approach helps people develop fundamental training skills and reduce the risk of training-related injuries.

Reversibility

The principle of reversibility refers to the fact that the adaptations to training will be lost when training ceases or is significantly reduced. Adaptations to training can be easily lost.

The time and effort put into training spark adaptations in muscle, heart, and other tissues that enable the body to tolerate increased levels of exercise intensity and duration. Those same adaptations will be lost or substantially diminished if training is reduced or discontinued (figure 5.2). However, during times of the year when it is not possible to sustain a full training program, a maintenance training program can preserve most of the adaptations.

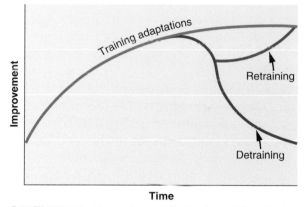

FIGURE 5.2 Detraining results in a loss of the adaptations to training, but with retraining, a trained person will adapt more quickly than an untrained person.

Research shows that gains in muscle strength can be maintained for about the first three weeks of detraining before loss in strength begins to accelerate.

Progressive Overload

The principle of progressive overload is the cornerstone of all training programs. To optimize the adaptations to training, the training load (the combination of intensity, duration, frequency, and mode) should be gradually increased to progressively overload the muscles, heart, and other tissues to provide enough stress to stimulate adaptations. Virtually any type of training that stresses the body beyond the level it has become accustomed to will result in adaptations that increase the body's capacity for exercise. The ever-present risk is that too much training will overwhelm the body's ability to adapt and create a condition of overtraining—the failure of the body to adapt, resulting in a significant reduction in training and performance capacity. In addition, overuse injuries such as shin splints and sore joints are common when the training load consistently exceeds the individual's capacity to adapt. A gradual increase in overall training load prompts the most improvement.

Variation

The principle of variation—also referred to as the principle of periodization—is the concept that varying the mode, intensity, duration, and frequency of training is effective at maintaining a training load that maximizes adaptations and minimizes the risk of overtraining. Varying the mode, intensity, duration, and frequency of training is required to maximize adaptations and minimize the risk of overtraining.

Coaches and personal trainers recognize that repeating the same type of training over and over leads to physical and psychological staleness and is counterproductive to maximizing training adaptations. For that reason, long-term training programs should include variations that maintain an appropriate training stress while varying mode, intensity, duration, and frequency. Periodization in a training program that includes macrocycles, mesocycles, and microcycles is an example of the principle of variation.

Block Periodization

Training periodization schemes are helpful in part because they require short- and long-term planning and goal setting. One challenge with periodized training is that so many goals can be established that the process becomes overwhelming, both physically and psychologically. This is particularly true with sport training (as opposed to fitness training) because sport training requires the development of many specific skills, complicating the design and execution of a periodized training program. An alternative approach is to include blocks of specialized training cycles that focus on just a few fitness characteristics or sport skills, creating mesocycles that build in logical order toward pre-established performance or fitness goals. In theory, block periodized training reduces the risk of overtraining that can occur as a result of trying to accomplish too much too soon. In addition, block periodization allows athletes and clients to narrow their training focus to fewer short-term goals, increasing the likelihood of noticeable improvements before moving on to the next training block.

Reference: Issurin, V.B. (2010). New horizons for the methodology and physiology of training periodization. *Sports Medicine, 40*(3):189-206.

What Makes an Effective Training Program?

Training to reach a goal would be easy if all you had to do is exercise a little harder today than you did yesterday. With each day you'd be in better shape than the day before. As long as you added more exercise stress with every passing day, your body would continually adapt and you'd get fitter and fitter. If only that were the case.

In figure 5.3, example A depicts the progress that would be made if you were able to improve every day. Example B illustrates the overtraining syndrome that usually occurs if you try to follow the pattern in example A: too much training too soon without adequate rest. Example C shows the stair-step approach of a progressive overload training program that includes periods of reduced workload, allowing the body regular opportunities to adapt to the stress of training before the training load is gradually increased.

There are many variations of progressive overload training programs, but all include alternating periods of increased and decreased workload. These cycles stress the body for a period of time (the stimulus, or overreaching) and then allow time for adaptations to occur (the response). Throughout each cycle, it is essential to build in ample rest, nutrition, and hydration (the facilitators) to optimize the desired adaptations and reduce the risk of overtraining.

FIGURE 5.3 Three hypothetical examples of eight-month training programs.

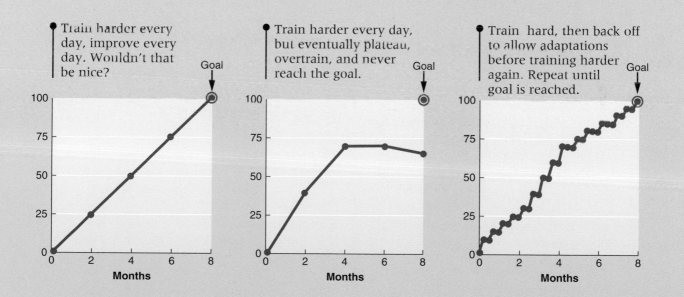

There is an endless variety of progressive overload training programs because each program has to take into consideration several factors. As an obvious example, a training program for football players in middle school will be quite different from a training program for college-aged football players. Likewise, a strength training program for a college-aged swimmer will be markedly different from that of a 44-year-old working mother who likes to swim for fitness. Table 5.1 summarizes the factors that have to be considered in the design of any training program. Answers to these 10 questions will help guide the creation of a training program that is tailored to meet the individual needs, interests, and goals of the athlete or client.

TABLE 5.1 **Questions on Program Design for Three Sample Clients**

Question	Anna	Dan	John
How old is the athlete or client?	32	26	55
What are the goals?	Complete an Olympic-distance triathlon.	Race a marathon.	Increase muscle mass and lose fat.
How much experience with sport or exercise?	Ran track for two years in high school. Periodic fitness classes in college and after graduation.	Track and cross country in high school; track scholarship in college.	Golf team in high school. Has run local road races; enjoys bicycling and lifting weights.
What are the skill levels?	Beginner in swimming and cycling. Some experience with run training.	Advanced. Ran the mile in college (4:02) and has read about marathon training programs.	Above-average and seems athletic. Has tried a lot of fitness routines.
Any injuries or health problems?	No. Had shin splints in high school track season.	None.	Periodic low back pain.
How committed to training?	Seems excited about trying something new and indicates that she will train on her own when needed.	Very committed. Overtraining may be a risk.	Willing to train before or after work.
What is the overall level of interest in the sport or activity?	Excited to be involved in triathlon because many of her friends are triathletes.	Would like to finish under 2:20.	Motivated by the desire to maintain strength and mass as he ages.
How competitive in both intent and skill?	Beginner in both regards. Too soon to tell if she will develop a competitive streak.	Extremely competitive. Has racing experience and knows how to train.	Competition is less important than changes in body composition and fitness.
How much time able and willing to devote to training?	Willing to train at least 3 days per week.	Willing to train 6 days each week.	Thinks he can train at least 4 days each week.
What are the deadlines for accomplishing key goals?	Sprint triathlon in 3 months. Olympic distance in 5 months.	First marathon in 4 months, next one in 6 months.	Would like to see changes in 4 to 6 weeks.

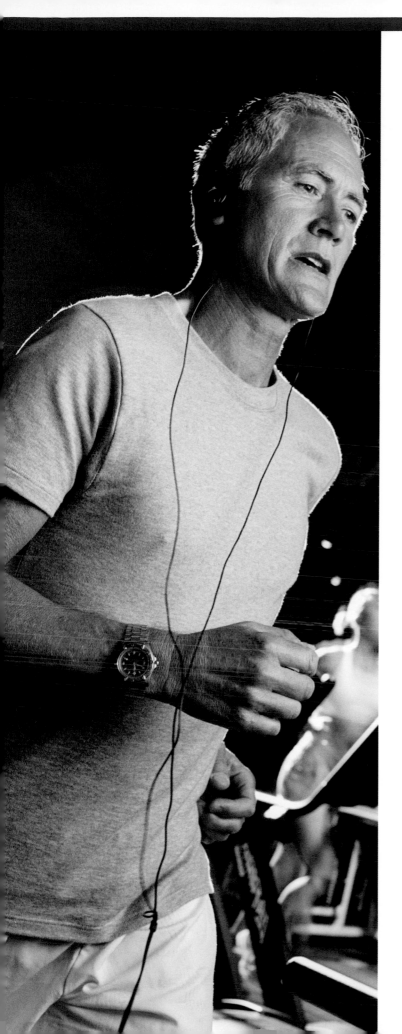

Adaptation Is the Goal

The word *adaptation* is used repeatedly throughout this book because the intent of training is to maximize adaptations in muscle and other tissues. To refresh your memory, all adaptations occur as a result of individual cells producing more functional proteins such as enzymes, signaling molecules, contractile proteins, and structural proteins. An increase in the functional protein content of cells increases their capacity to meet the demands of exercise. Here are three examples:

❶ In liver cells, adaptations in functional proteins increase the liver's capacity to store glycogen that can be used to maintain blood glucose concentrations during exercise.

❷ In skeletal muscle cells, adaptations in functional proteins increase the cell's capacity to produce ATP faster and for a longer time (among many other adaptations).

❸ In cells of the blood vessels, adaptations in functional proteins enable the vessels to better dilate and constrict to meet the changing demands for blood flow that occur during exercise.

Overreaching Is a Good Thing, but Overtraining Is Not

All adaptations in functional proteins within cells occur in response to *overreaching* during training, pushing the body so that it naturally adapts to increasing levels of exercise stress. A central challenge in designing any training program is to ensure that overreaching does not result in overtraining. One way to accomplish that goal is to follow the *principle of progressive overload,* as illustrated in figure 5.4.

The example in figure 5.4 shows how an eight-month training program with a specific goal (that could be a weight-loss goal, a strength-related goal, a performance goal, a MET-related goal, and so on) can be broken down into training segments, or *cycles.* In this example, two four-month *macrocycles* allow for subgoals to be established so that progress toward the ultimate goal can be assessed along the way. That same approach also applies to the two-month *mesocycles* and the two-week *microcycles.* Dividing a training program into separate parts allows for each part to be designed to accomplish specific fitness goals that progressively build toward the ultimate goal. If sufficient progress is not made within a microcycle, then subsequent training can be altered to ensure that future subgoals can be met.

FIGURE 5.4 An example of an eight-month training program that incorporates macrocycles, mesocycles, and microcycles, each of which has its own goals for exercise mode, intensity, duration, frequency, and rest.

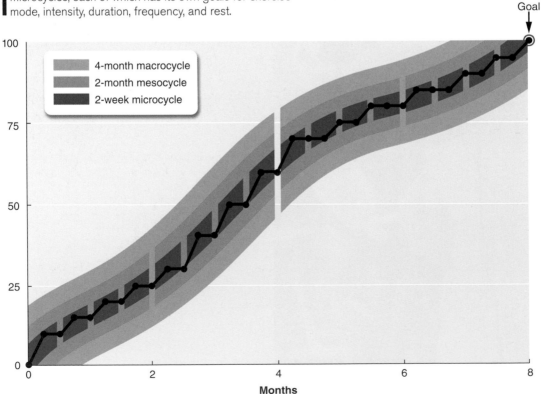

For example, if a 42-year-old woman who has run in a few local 5K road races (3.1 miles) wants to train for a half-marathon event (13.1 miles) eight months from now, the goal of each monthly microcycle could be to increase her weekly training mileage in increments so that she reaches 25 to 30 miles per week in the seventh microcycle before tapering her mileage during the final microcycle leading up to the race. The goal of each two-month mesocycle could be to gradually increase her average running pace, and the goal of the four-month macrocycles could be to lower her 5K run times by at least 10%. Obviously there are many ways to structure micro-, meso-, and macrocycles to construct short- and long-term goals to guide training and at the same time create motivational markers that keep athletes and clients psychologically challenged and excited.

Notice in figure 5.4 that every increase in training capacity (the sloped blue lines) is followed by a period in which training workload plateaus (or in some cases may even decrease). Periodically lowering the training workload for a few days or even longer allows time for adaptations in functional proteins while reducing the risk of overtraining. Keep in mind that figure 5.4 is simply *one* example of how the principle of progressive overload can be integrated into a training program that incorporates macro-, meso-, and microcycles. In addition to having varied goals and modes of training, programs might be of varying lengths with different lengths and numbers of macro-, meso-, and microcycles.

Before important competitions, the training load should be gradually reduced to help maximize the various adaptations to training. This reduction in training load is commonly referred to as *tapering*. Research with swimmers, runners, and cyclists indicates that the optimal tapering strategy is accomplished over the two weeks before an important competition by decreasing the training volume by 40% to 60% without changing training intensity or frequency. Using the half-marathon runner as an example, her training mileage in the last two weeks might decrease from 30 miles per week to 15 miles per week, but she would maintain the number of days she trained each week (frequency) and her running pace (intensity).

> Overtrained athletes have reductions in maximal oxygen uptake, cardiac output, systolic blood pressure, and circulating epinephrine (adrenaline) levels.

A Little More About Overtraining

Most athletes and clients are motivated to work hard to achieve their goals. Sometimes that diligence goes too far, resulting in overtraining (also called the *overtraining syndrome*). Overtraining is bad news because it can't be corrected with just a few days of rest. Sometimes athletes need six months or more of rest in order to resolve all the symptoms of overtraining, a depressing, frustrating, and trying time. With that bleak scenario in mind, you need to understand overtraining so that you can help prevent it.

As described in chapter 4, the symptoms of overtraining include reduced strength, coordination, and endurance; loss of motivation and enjoyment; depression; loss of appetite; weight loss; sleep disturbance, irritability and lack of focus; and changes in heart rate and blood pressure. Overtraining is the result of complex interactions that occur among the nervous, endocrine, immune, and musculoskeletal systems.

Overtraining is a failure to adapt. Even worse, the athlete's performance doesn't just plateau; it deteriorates. Unfortunately, there is no reliable blood test to warn of impending overtraining. However, the good news is that periodically monitoring exercise heart rate during a standardized exercise task does seem to be an effective way to predict the possibility of overtraining and therefore the need for a few days of rest. Experienced trainers and coaches can often tell when a client or athlete begins to overtrain by noting negative changes in disposition, enthusiasm for training, and particularly training capacity. Sometimes it is difficult to convince an athlete to back off training, but doing so may be the only way to prevent overtraining syndrome.

Some of the Causes of Overtraining Include

Alterations in

- Brain neurotransmitters
- Brain structures
- Motor nerve function
- Hormonal response
- Immune response
- Muscle function

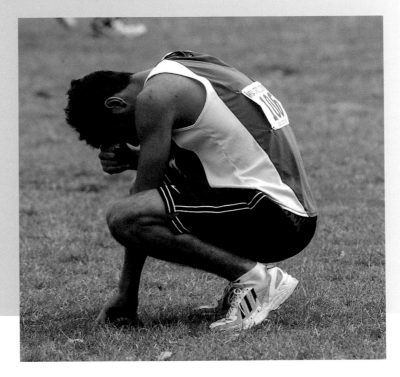

Training Terms

Few things are more boring than a list of glossary terms, but in this case it's important that you know the pertinent terminology and meanings. For example, if an athlete asks you for advice on becoming more agile, it's essential that you both agree on the definition of *agility* so that your understanding and her expectations are clear. So, with that simple goal in mind, following are formal definitions of a few terms and some examples of statements containing those terms.

adaptation—The process by which various changes in the body enable it to adjust to a new environment or condition. "Exercise training stimulates *adaptations* in muscle cells that improve the cells' ability to produce the energy needed for improved performance."

agility—The ability to change directions quickly and accurately. "She has really helped our team this year because her *agility* on defense has improved."

duration—The length of time in which an event occurs. "In the next training session, we'll increase your workload by increasing the *duration* of your repeat sprints."

endurance—The ability to resist fatigue, as in muscular endurance or cardio-respiratory endurance. "To improve your performance in the fourth quarter, you have to improve your *endurance*."

fatigue—The inability to continue a task, often associated with temporary feelings of tiredness. "For maximal muscle adaptation, it's important that you periodically exercise to *fatigue*."

intensity—The magnitude of effort. "Increasing the *intensity* of your repeat sprints will improve your anaerobic as well as your aerobic fitness."

mode—A particular form or variety of something. "We'll frequently change the *mode* of exercise to keep your mind and body from getting too accustomed to doing the same thing."

overload—A greater-than-normal training stress or load. "For your muscles to adapt properly, you have to *overload* them periodically."

overreaching—A planned and systematic attempt to stress the body beyond its normal capacity. "Every effective training program incorporates the concept of *overreaching* followed by periods of reduced training workload or rest."

overtraining—Regularly doing more work than can be physically tolerated. "That team usually does poorly during the season because their coach doesn't understand the difference between overreaching and *overtraining*."

overtraining syndrome—Failure of the body to adapt to exercise training characterized by weeks or months of deteriorating performance and training capacity. "She has suffered from *overtraining syndrome* during each of the past two seasons because her coach insists that she train every day."

periodization—Division into periods. "An effective way to progressively overload the athlete's body is to use a *periodization* approach to designing the training program.

power—An index of the rate at which work can be done. Power applies similarly to athletes, racehorses, and engines. Improvements in performance often require an increase in power. "A football linebacker can increase his *power* simply by losing body fat."

repetitions (reps)—The act of repeating a function. "We'll gradually increase the number of *reps* on the bench press as you become stronger."

sets—A group of repetitions (reps). "Research shows that three *sets* of 8 to 12 reps seem to optimize gains in strength."

speed—The rate of movement. In mathematical terms, speed is the distance traveled divided by the time of travel. "We can create a training program to improve your *speed* in the 40-yard sprint."

strength—The ability of a muscle to exert force. "The correct kind of resistance exercise will help older adults improve their grip *strength*, making everyday tasks easier."

tapering—Reducing the training load before important competitions in an attempt to maximize performance. "With the state championships only three weeks away, we're almost ready to start our *tapering*."

training variables—The components of a training program that can be manipulated: intensity, duration, mode, and frequency. "Our training program incorporates gradual changes in *training variables* so that our clients overreach without becoming overtrained."

training volume—The composite of training variables. "You can increase your *training volume* by increasing training frequency, duration, and intensity either individually or in combination."

work—In mathematical terms, force multiplied by distance. "You accomplish *work* whenever you walk up a flight of stairs."

workload—The amount of work expected, assigned, or accomplished. "You've really improved these last few weeks, so next week we'll increase your *workload*."

CHAPTER SIX

Training to Improve Muscle Mass and Strength

Muscles respond rapidly to resistance training by recruiting more motor units and laying down new muscle proteins, a response that is affected by diet.

In this photo, you can see the bulging biceps muscle straining against the barbell, with forearm muscles also engaged to lock the wrist in place. Nerve impulses from the brain have activated motor units in the arm flexor muscles and in a variety of muscles in the torso and legs for stabilization. The man in the photo could likely complete many repetitions with this weight before fatiguing. If his goal is to build biceps strength and mass, how many sets and reps should he complete? How much weight should he lift? How many times each week? With strength training, when is the point of diminishing return? In other words, is strength training for an hour five times each week any better at building strength and mass than training in just one or two shorter sessions each week?

Techniques for increasing muscle strength have been a central part of sport training for centuries, so you'd think that by this time sport scientists and trainers would have a clear idea of what works best for building strength and mass. They don't. In fact, there is healthy ongoing debate about how much and how often people should engage in strength training to optimize the cellular adaptations that lead to increased strength and greater muscle mass. That debate is fueled by inconsistent research findings. To begin this chapter, revisit the physiological changes that are needed for increased strength and mass.

How Do Strength and Mass Increase?

As you remember from chapter 1, several adaptations to strength training occur in the central nervous system and in the muscle cells.

In people who are new to strength training or haven't engaged in strength training for a few months or longer, muscle strength increases soon after training begins. That increase in strength has nothing to do with an increase in contractile proteins and everything to do with increased recruitment of motor units. As the nervous system recruits more motor units, force production (strength) increases because more muscle cells are involved in each contraction. With time, muscle cells adapt to the continuing stress of strength training by creating more proteins (actin, myosin, troponin, tropomyosin, titin, and many others), and muscle mass increases. How much muscle mass is added as a result of strength training depends on the factors shown in figure 6.1.

The most obvious influence on the amount of muscle mass developed as a result of strength training is genetics. It's obvious that some people do not have the genetic predisposition to add large amounts of muscle mass, whereas others do. The extent to which a person can add muscle mass is primarily determined by genotype (inherited genetic makeup), which establishes an upper limit of sorts for muscle mass and all other characteristics of cells, a good example of how nature determines what nurture can accomplish. However, everyone can add mass and increase muscle strength with the proper training program. That's because phenotype is determined by the interaction of genotype and environment. In the case of muscle mass, environment includes factors such as extent of physical activity in childhood, age of starting strength training, duration of strength training, diet, and current methods of strength training. Age and sex also play roles.

Training of any sort alters phenotype, at least until training ceases and the adaptations disappear. The stimulus of strength training is intended to provoke an adaptive response: the addition of proteins to muscle cells that enable greater force production as well as an increase in the size of individual cells and consequently the entire muscle. Strength training triggers signals within the muscle cell that stimulate the nuclei to churn out more contractile proteins that are then added to the cell. In other words, effective strength training causes an increase in muscle protein syn-thesis, proteins produced through the interaction of the cell's signaling molecules with the DNA in the many nuclei within each muscle cell. Genotype determines how responsive muscle nuclei will be to strength training and therefore how many new muscle proteins will be added before reaching the upper limit imposed by genotype.

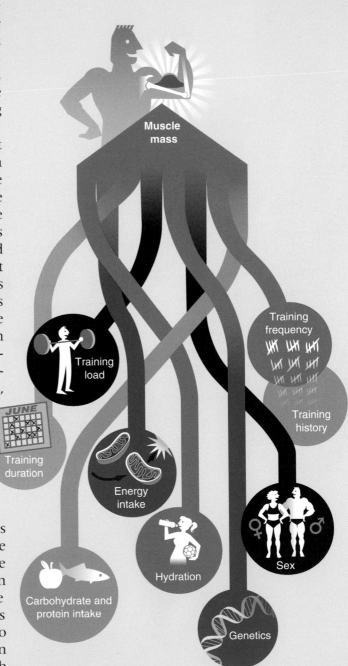

FIGURE 6.1 Factors that influence muscle mass.

Adaptations to Strength Training

- More motor units recruited
- Greater stimulation frequency of motor units
- More synchronous recruiting of motor units
- Reduced inhibition of motor units
- Increased size of muscle cells (hypertrophy)
- Possibly a small increase in number of muscle cells (hyperplasia)
- Increased bone mineral density and bone strength
- Increased strength of ligaments and tendons

Causes of Hypertrophy

- More contractile proteins (actin and myosin)
- More structural proteins
- More sarcoplasm
- More myofibril units
- More connective tissue
- More intracellular water
- More muscle cells (maybe)

Can Women Increase Strength Without Dramatically Increasing Muscle Mass?

The simple answer is yes. Remember that significant gains in muscle strength occur early in training before muscle mass has a chance to increase. Those strength gains are associated with the recruitment of more motor units. Women who want to gain strength and improve muscle function but do not want to develop large muscles can train with lighter weights and tailor their long-term training program accordingly. Strength training results in larger muscles, but the extent of the increase in muscle size is determined by genetics and the type of strength training. Another important factor in determining how much muscle mass is added as a result of training is testosterone production. Testosterone is an anabolic and androgen steroid hormone. In other words, testosterone promotes anabolic responses such as the gain in mass and strength that accompanies resistance training as well as androgenic responses such as the growth of body hair and lower voice that accompany puberty in boys. Estrogen, the primary sex hormone in females, is produced directly from testosterone. For that reason, all females produce testosterone in small quantities. As a result, the anabolic responses to strength training in women are muted compared to the responses in men, who benefit from higher testosterone levels. Estrogen is produced in the ovaries and fat cells from testosterone, which is produced from cholesterol. The impact of estrogen on muscles and connective tissues in response to training is not well understood.

This program shows an example of how strength training workouts can be customized to match the goals of the athlete or client. This example illustrates how training for three 32-year-old women can be modified to meet their varying interests and goals.

Level	Goal	Upper-back muscles	Quadriceps muscles
32-year-old female beginner	Transition from sedentary to active lifestyle Improve muscle tone Lose fat mass	Lat pull-down machine Seated row machine Reverse fly with light tension band	Leg press Body-weight step-up Leg extension
		3 sets of 15 to 20 repetitions **Moderate weight with 60 to 90 sec rest**	
32-year-old female fitness enthusiast	Increase muscle strength. Better-defined muscles without adding too much lean mass Increase stamina for fitness classes	Assisted chin-up Dumbbell row Cable crossover reverse fly	Barbell back squat Weighted reverse lunge Lunge jump
		3 sets of 12 to 15 reps **Moderate to heavy weight with 30 to 45 sec rest**	
32-year-old female competitive athlete	Increase strength for triathlon performance Willing to gain some lean mass	Body-weight chin-up* Dumbbell prone lying pullover Single-arm low cable row with rotation	Barbell front squat Weighted step-up with reverse lunge Med-ball squat jump
		3 sets of 10 to 12 **Moderate to heavy weight with 90 to 120 sec rest** ***Work to failure, then perform 3 successive negative reps**	

Workouts were created by Kelly Schnell, BS, CSCS, ACSM-CPT.

What's the Best Way to Gain Strength and Mass?

Muscles are very plastic. No, muscles aren't *made* of plastic, but muscles do have a remarkable ability to adapt very quickly to varying conditions, a feature known as *plasticity*. Muscles start adapting within days of training and, on the other end of the spectrum, begin to lose those adaptations within days of no training. When a limb is put in a cast or when a person is confined to bed for long periods, muscles atrophy—that is, they experience a marked reduction in protein and lose size and strength, changes that can be reversed with training. This section focuses on muscle hypertrophy and the best way to add muscle mass and strength.

You have already learned that muscle cells increase their content of functional proteins in response to training, adaptations that allow the cells to increase their capacity for doing work. This increase in functional protein content continues for as long as the muscles are progressively overloaded, eventually plateauing at a limit set by genotype. Too much strength training too soon not only increases the risk of injury but also leads to overreaching and perhaps overtraining, conditions discussed in chapter 5 that reduce the production of functional proteins. Just the right amount of training leads to progressive increases in strength and mass. So what is just the right amount of strength training? How many sets? How many reps? How often?

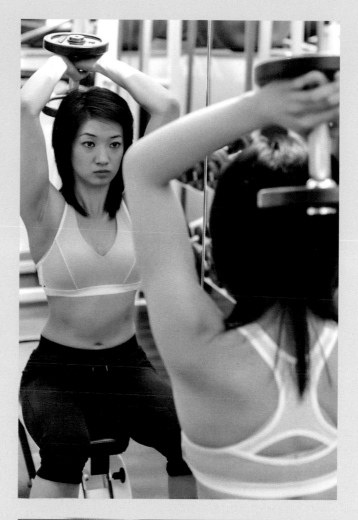

Strength training exposes muscles to a variety of stimuli that interact to produce an increase in muscle protein synthesis. Those stimuli include mechanical stress on muscle cells; increased motor unit recruitment; swelling of active muscle cells; the postworkout increase in hormones such as testosterone, growth hormone, and insulinlike growth factor (IGF-1); the accumulation of metabolites such as lactic acid; and the increased production of free radicals (e.g., reactive oxygen species). All of these stimuli interact to determine the overall increase in muscle protein synthesis.

General Guidelines for
Resistance Training Programs

Based on the available research, here are some practical tips around which strength training programs should be designed. These principles apply regardless of the goal of the strength training program, be it for someone starting a fitness program, an athlete seeking to improve sport-specific strength, or a bodybuilder striving to add muscle mass. Of course, a caveat is that everyone should first learn proper exercise technique and have ample time to experience the training program at low intensities before learning how to exercise to failure. Endless variations in strength training programs can be developed around these principles, so these tips should be considered the building blocks for designing and individualizing strength training.

▌ **Once or twice a week.** More strength training is not better and therefore not needed. That does not mean that people can't or shouldn't strength-train more frequently if they choose. It does mean that training individual muscle groups more than twice each week will not produce dramatically greater gains in strength and mass. In other words, a strength training program that works arms, shoulders, chest, and back on Mondays and Wednesdays, and abs, glutes, and legs on Tuesdays and Thursdays adheres to the two-days-per-week maximum.

▌ **One set, 8 to 12 reps.** The secret is to reach *temporary muscle failure* with each set. Lifting a weight heavy enough to cause muscles to fatigue after just 8 to 12 repetitions provides a maximal training stimulus that will lead to maximal adaptations. More sets or more reps do nothing to add strength or mass. Doing at least one warm-up set before each max set is a smart way to reduce risk of injury and get in the frame of mind needed for the max set. Once 12 reps are exceeded in the max set, it's time to increase the resistance. Of course, heavy resistance isn't for everyone, so if multiple sets with more than 12 reps are needed, that too will lead to gains in strength and mass, provided that the muscle groups are consistently exercised to failure. It will just take more time in each workout to get there. For example, a strength training program for a football lineman might include 3 sets of 8 reps with heavy resistance, while a defensive back on the same team might complete a warm-up and then 1 or 2 sets of 20 reps with lighter resistance but faster contractions. See table 6.1 for an example of a 20-minute strength training workout for increasing strength and mass.

▌ **Stay steady.** Keep all movements smooth and steady in both directions to maximally stress the muscles. Lifting too rapidly creates momentum that reduces the overall stress on the muscle and increases the risk of injury.

▌ **Equipment doesn't matter.** Use whatever equipment is available; just make sure to exercise to momentary failure. There is no doubt that some types of exercise equipment have advantages in terms of comfort, stability, range of motion, joint forces, equipment footprint, and other factors, but fancy equipment is not needed for building strength. If you doubt that, arm-wrestle a farmer sometime.

▌ **One limb at a time.** Whether it's a chest press, a biceps curl, or a squat, training only one arm or leg at a time requires engagement of the core muscles for stabilization. That means multiple muscle groups get a workout, and that is a good thing for overall strength development.

❚ **Mix it up.** There is no need to repeat the same exercises for months on end. As long as muscles are exercised to momentary fatigue, increases in strength and mass will occur.

❚ **Your parents are the ones to blame (or thank).** Your genotype determines how you respond to exercise, and strength training is no exception. Those who quickly become stronger and more toned have their parents to thank. Those who work harder than everyone else and see only a fraction of the improvement have their parents to blame.

❚ **Protein is your friend.** So are water and carbohydrate. A hydrated muscle is an anabolic muscle, so staying hydrated throughout the day promotes muscle anabolism. After a workout, tired muscles need carbohydrate to replenish their energy stores and protein to jump-start muscle repair and growth. Normal meals and snacks provide those nutrients, but consuming a large glass of chocolate milk or similar protein drink immediately after a workout will supply muscles with the protein and carbohydrate needed for optimizing recovery and growth.

Time crunch? Table 6.1 is a sample program based on the principles explained previously that provides an effective full-body workout in only 20 minutes. The only equipment needed is a set of dumbbells. In this workout, transition immediately from one exercise to the next, and increase the resistance once you achieve 12 reps in the max set. Emphasize proper form and use a spotter when needed.

The highest rate of muscle growth in response to strength training is about 1% per week.

TABLE 6.1 **20-Minute Workout for Strength and Mass**

Exercise	Warm-up set	Max set
Right-arm curl	1 set of 10 reps, light weight	1 set of 8 to 12 reps, heavy weight
Left-arm row	1 set of 10 reps, light weight	1 set of 8 to 12 reps, heavy weight
Abs (plank, crunch)	30 sec	30 sec
Right-arm triceps kickback	1 set of 10 reps, light weight	1 set of 8 to 12 reps, heavy weight
Left-arm chest press	1 set of 10 reps, light weight	1 set of 8 to 12 reps, heavy weight
Abs (plank, crunch)	30 sec	30 sec
Left-leg squat	1 set of 10 reps, light weight	1 set of 8 to 12 reps, heavy weight
Right-arm chest press	1 set of 10 reps, light weight	1 set of 8 to 12 reps, heavy weight
Abs (plank, crunch)	30 sec	30 sec
Left-arm triceps kickback	1 set of 10 reps, light weight	1 set of 8 to 12 reps, heavy weight
Right-arm row	1 set of 10 reps, light weight	1 set of 8 to 12 reps, heavy weight
Abs (plank, crunch)	30 sec	30 sec
Left-arm curl	1 set of 10 reps, light weight	1 set of 8 to 12 reps, heavy weight
Right-leg squat	1 set of 10 reps, light weight	1 set of 8 to 12 reps, heavy weight

How Do Anabolic Steroids Work?

It didn't take unscrupulous athletes, coaches, scientists, and physicians long to figure out that the natural limits imposed by genotype could be exceeded with pharmacology. Most anabolic steroids that athletes use to improve performance are substances that mimic the effects of testosterone. In addition to the natural precursors of testosterone such as DHEA and androstenedione, numerous designer steroids are illicitly produced in laboratories by making small alterations to the structure of the testosterone molecule. Other anabolic molecules such as insulin, growth hormone (GH), and insulinlike growth factor (IGF) are essential hormones that support many normal bodily functions by stimulating the nuclei in cells to produce proteins such as enzymes, signaling molecules, structural proteins, and contractile proteins. When muscle cells are exposed to higher-than-normal levels of anabolic hormones, peptides, and growth factors, the cell nuclei produce more proteins, adding to the protein-producing stimulus created by strength training.

Steroids stimulate muscle cell nuclei to produce more contractile proteins, adding to the stimulus created by strength training.

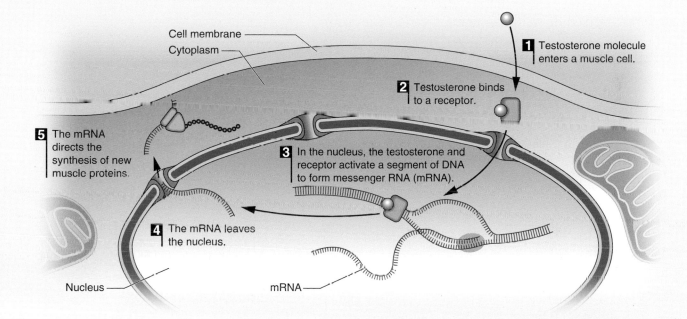

Cell membrane
Cytoplasm

1 Testosterone molecule enters a muscle cell.

2 Testosterone binds to a receptor.

5 The mRNA directs the synthesis of new muscle proteins.

3 In the nucleus, the testosterone and receptor activate a segment of DNA to form messenger RNA (mRNA).

4 The mRNA leaves the nucleus.

Nucleus

mRNA

Using anabolic steroids (testosterone and its natural precursors or synthetic analogues) to augment performance is clearly cheating because doping creates an unfair competitive advantage. In addition, using anabolic steroids is associated with a variety of health risks that include liver damage, enlarged prostate glands, reduced stature (among young athletes), testicular atrophy, reduced sperm count, enlarged male breasts (termed *gynecomastia*), acne, masculinization of females, disrupted menstruation, growth of facial hair, breast atrophy, and deepening of the voice. Long-term use of growth hormone is associated with cardiomyopathy, acromegaly (enlarged skull), hypertension, heart disease, and weakening of joints and connective tissue. These negative consequences should not be surprising, because disrupting the intricate control of hormonal function by indiscriminate doping is bound to disrupt normal cellular function.

How Important Is the Type of Muscle Contraction?

When it comes to strength training, variety is a good thing. It's psychologically refreshing to be faced with a new challenge periodically along with different equipment and exercise variation to stress muscles in different ways. Free weights, machine weights, elastic bands, stability balls, kettlebells, weighted balls, and other equipment all have a legitimate place in a strength training program (see figure 6.2).

It is important to remember that muscle cells can contract in various ways that affect overall force production. For example, the concentric contractions needed to lift a weight require that muscle cells shorten, with actin and myosin filaments sliding over one another, creating a bulging muscle with each repetition. When that weight is slowly lowered, the muscle cells lengthen (eccentric contraction) while still producing force as the actin and myosin filaments continue to interact and the elastic connective tissue of the muscle is stretched, contributing to force production. In isometric contractions, the joint is held in a fixed position while muscle cells shorten and then maintain a sustained contraction. Most sports require a dynamic, ever-changing combination of all three types of contractions, and strength training programs can include exercises that mimic those conditions. The use of unstable surfaces such as balance boards and vibration platforms adds more psychological challenge and physical stress to exercises. This challenge may augment strength development and adds interest and variety to a training program.

Eccentric exercises are particularly effective at building strength and mass because heavier weights can be used. Heavier weights mean greater stress on the muscle, and that translates into stronger signals for production of functional proteins. However, because of the increased stress on the muscle, eccentric exercises are associated with greater DOMS (delayed-onset muscle soreness) and risk of injury. In addition, many eccentric exercises require special equipment or a trained spotter to help with the workout. In practical terms, improvements in strength and mass depend more on a person's dedication to the training program than on a particular piece of equipment or exercise routine. There are many ways to increase muscle strength and mass, and you should keep that simple fact in mind when developing strength training programs.

The response to strength training is an increase in the production of prostaglandins, molecules that influence the overall response to training. The primary enzyme responsible for prostaglandin production is cyclooxygenase (COX). COX activity is inhibited by nonsteroidal anti-inflammatory drugs (NSAIDs) such as acetaminophen, ibuprofen, and aspirin, leading to the concern that consuming NSAIDs on a regular basis—as many athletes do—might reduce the benefits of strength training. Fortunately, research indicates that NSAID use at normal doses does not seem to negatively influence the development of muscle strength and mass.

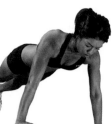

Push-ups involve both concentric (dynamic) and eccentric muscle contractions: concentric on the way up, eccentric on the way down.

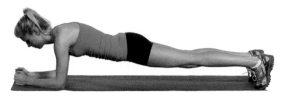

A plank is an example of isometric (static) muscle contractions involving many muscle groups.

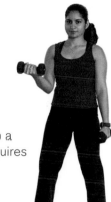

Any exercise in which a weight is lowered requires muscles to contract eccentrically.

Kettlebell weights can create resistance for concentric, eccentric, and isometric contractions.

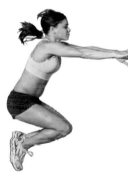

Plyometric exercises require concentric and eccentric muscle contractions.

Stability balls and weighted balls can load muscles in different ways.

Strength training machines and free weights are similarly effective at building strength and mass as long as muscles are stressed appropriately.

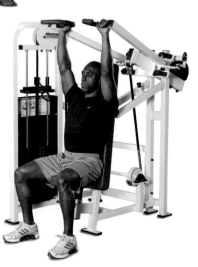

FIGURE 6.2 Various types of equipment and muscle contractions create variety and stress muscles in different ways.

Strength Training Gimmicks . . . or Not?

Everyone involved in strength training would like to find a competitive edge—a quicker way to develop strength and mass. Endless ads in magazines and online tout shortcuts to superior strength with claims not necessarily based on superior science. Here are three examples:

❶ Electrical stimulation. The idea behind this technique is that if muscles can be stimulated to contract through electrodes placed on the skin, it could augment or replace strength training. Electrical stimulation is widely used in patients whose limbs are immobilized by casts after injury or surgery with the purpose of reducing the loss of strength and mass. However, there is no good evidence that electrical stimulation of muscles will increase strength or mass, because the stimulation generally produces submaximal contractions, an inadequate stimulus compared to a well-designed strength training routine. In theory, if electrical stimulation were used to produce a supramaximal contraction during strength training, it might induce greater gains in strength and mass. That sounds good in theory, but the practical downside is that the pain, muscle damage, and potential for injury associated with supramaximal electrical stimulation far outweigh the benefits.

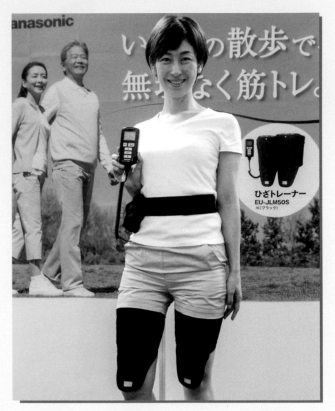

❷ Restricted blood flow. Another way to increase the stimulus to muscles during strength training is to restrict blood flow to the muscles, reducing the delivery of oxygen and nutrients as well as the removal of waste products. For those who cannot lift heavy weights (e.g., 80% of 1RM) because of age, illness, or injury, using a pressure cuff to reduce blood flow while lifting light weights (e.g., 30% of 1RM) can theoretically increase the stimulus and produce greater gains in strength and mass. Reducing the blood flow to muscles during strength training may also stimulate the recruitment of motor units that are not usually involved in training, thereby enhancing the training effect. In fact, research indicates that occlusion training with light weight does result in increased strength and mass, a real benefit for those who are restricted in their ability to lift heavier weights. Restricting blood flow in healthy individuals might provide some variety in training, but the real benefit appears to be for people who are limited in one way or another in their ability to participate in conventional strength training.

❸ Compression clothing. Clothing designed to compress muscle groups such as the thigh and calf muscles has been developed to aid muscle function in training and competition. The premise is that the right amount of compression can improve blood flow through the muscles, stabilize muscle groups, and perhaps add an element of elasticity to augment jumping, sprinting, and other explosive movements. Research on sport compression clothing has produced mixed results, with most studies reporting no benefits to performance or recovery. However, no one has ever been harmed by sport compression clothing, so if the garment feels good to wear, that alone might be enough of a benefit to justify the cost of the clothing.

What's the Role of Nutrition?

Those interested in increasing strength and mass are often interested in how nutrition—especially protein nutrition—can help. This is an interesting area of sport science, and the research is clear that consuming high-quality protein after a workout will optimize muscle protein synthesis. From a practical perspective, that means consuming protein soon after a workout. The body digests protein into a variety of amino acids that are absorbed into the bloodstream. High-quality protein contains all the essential amino acids—most important the amino acid leucine and others the body cannot make—that muscles need to increase the synthesis of proteins such as the contractile, structural, transport, and regulatory proteins required for increased strength and mass. During workouts, muscle protein breakdown increases, which is a natural response to exercise. After workouts, it makes sense to reduce protein breakdown and increase protein synthesis to help speed muscle recovery, repair, and growth. Doing so on a regular basis accelerates increases in strength and mass. It also makes sense to consume protein snacks periodically during the day to bump up protein synthesis to further support the production of functional proteins in muscle.

Research demonstrates that 20 grams of high-quality protein found in milk, meat, eggs, and fish seems sufficient to maximally stimulate muscle protein synthesis after exercise. Older people (i.e., >50 years) demonstrate what researchers have termed *anabolic resistance* to protein intake in that they require 40 grams of protein for maximal stimulation of protein synthesis. The combination of exercise and protein intake is particularly important with aging because it helps

Food Servings That Contain 20 Grams of High-Quality Protein

5 egg whites (95 kcal)

3 ounces (85 g) turkey (90 kcal)

3 ounces (85 g) canned tuna (85 kcal)

3 ounces (85 g) chicken (90 kcal)

4.5 ounces (125 g) ham (125 kcal)

3.5 ounces (105 g) lean beef (130 kcal)

6 ounces (180 g) cottage cheese (160 kcal)

4 ounces (115 g) ground beef (200 kcal)

2.6 ounces (76 g) seitan (110 kcal)

protect against the loss of muscle mass, contributes to bone health, and aids in appetite control. A related benefit is that research shows that the stronger tend to live longer.

There is growing evidence that distributing protein intake evenly throughout the day, including before bedtime, will maximize muscle protein synthesis and help maintain or increase muscle mass. For example, a 180-pound (82 kg) athlete should consume roughly 1.5 grams of protein per kilogram of body weight each day. That's approximately 120 grams of protein per day that can be divided into four portions, each containing 30 grams of protein, perhaps as part of three regular meals and a snack before bedtime. Consuming protein in that manner has been shown to sustain higher rates of muscle protein synthesis.

Any time you complete a hard workout, there are surges in a variety of hormones in the bloodstream, part of the natural response to exercise. In addition, any time you eat a snack or meal, a hormonal response accompanies the ingestion of foods and beverages. Advertisements for some dietary supplements contain claims that the supplement provokes an increase in anabolic hormones that help increase strength and mass. If only it were that simple! Research shows that the hormonal response to resistance training and to the ingestion of dietary supplements does not play a critical role in developing strength and mass. There's no doubt that the hormonal response to exercise and diet is important, but so many other factors that occur in the days, weeks, and months of a training program have a far greater effect in the development of strength and mass.

One supplement that does seem to help improve strength and mass—at least in some people—is creatine monohydrate. Studies have reported a 10% to 20% increase in muscle phosphocreatine content and improvement in some tests of strength, power, and mass with creatine supplementation. Ingesting 5 grams of creatine monohydrate each day for a month has been shown to be effective at increasing muscle phosphocreatine content. A loading dose of 20 grams per day for five days has a similar effect. Creatine supplementation has few side effects (e.g., upset stomach on the higher loading doses) but, to err on the side of caution, is not recommended for those who have kidney disease or are predisposed to kidney disease (e.g., people with diabetes).

CHAPTER SEVEN

Training for Weight Loss

Here's why moving more and eating less is great advice.

At any given time, at least a thousand diets of various sorts are touted to promote rapid weight loss. Add to that confusing scenario countless advertisements for dietary supplements that promise the same and then layer on weekly news flashes about the latest scientific discoveries that promise to ignite the body's fat-burning machinery, and that's just a glimpse of the information overload awaiting anyone interested in losing weight. Fortunately, the principles of effective weight loss—losing excess body fat and keeping it off—are not as complicated as they might appear. Changes in body weight—either up or down—occur because of changes in energy balance.

Weight Loss Is All About Energy Balance

You might recall from chapter 2 that energy is the capacity to do work. That work could be related to the contraction of a skeletal muscle cell, the transport of glucose across a membrane, the creation of an intracellular signal, or the synthesis of a functional protein such as an enzyme. All of that work requires ATP. And ATP production requires the oxidation of glucose and fat.

Converting the energy in a glucose molecule or a fatty-acid molecule into ATP is inefficient; 60% of the energy in glucose and fat is lost as heat during the production of ATP. That inefficiency is not all bad, though, because that heat helps keep body temperature normal.

The *first law of thermodynamics* (don't go to sleep quite yet!) indicates that energy is not created or destroyed; it simply changes from one form to another. As an example, the chemical energy in a glucose molecule is changed into the chemical energy in an ATP molecule that is changed into the mechanical energy of a muscle contraction that is changed into the kinetic energy of a body movement. No energy has been created and none has been destroyed. In fact, all of the energy associated with human movement is due to the energy of the sun (review the beginning of chapter 2 if you need a quick refresher). The energy in the sun's radiation is transformed by plants into chemical energy (e.g., starch and sugar). We and other animals consume plants (and we consume some of the animals) and thereby capture their chemical energy in the form of carbohydrate, fat, and protein.

The concept of *energy balance* is simple and irrefutable yet maddeningly complicated in its application to weight loss. For now, stick with the simple part. When energy intake is the same as energy output (energy expenditure), the total amount of energy in the body remains unchanged (see figure 7.1). In other words, body weight remains unchanged.

• When energy intake is greater than energy output, the total energy content of the body increases, as does body weight.

• Just the opposite happens when energy intake is less than energy output: The total energy content of the body falls and so does weight.

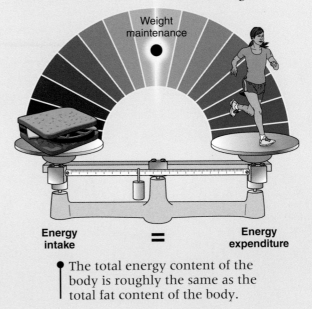

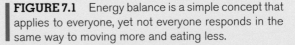

Energy intake **=** Energy expenditure

• The total energy content of the body is roughly the same as the total fat content of the body.

FIGURE 7.1 Energy balance is a simple concept that applies to everyone, yet not everyone responds in the same way to moving more and eating less.

Here is a closer look at both sides of the energy balance equation. On the energy intake side, the key factor is the amount of energy ingested as food and beverages. That energy is measured as Calories (kilocalories, or kcal), and energy intake actually means Calorie intake. Of course, many factors other than energy expenditure influence energy intake, such as the availability of food, serving sizes, hunger and satiety hormones, and emotional connections with eating.

On the energy output side of the equation, the number of Calories you expend in a day is determined by an equally large number of factors. Fortunately, that large number can be reduced to four easy-to-understand categories: resting metabolic rate, thermic effect of food, energy efficiency, and physical activity energy expenditure (see figure 7.2).

Overeating can lead to increased thermogenesis (heat production) because muscle and other cells increase fat oxidation and energy expenditure. Unfortunately, that thermogenesis cannot increase sufficiently to offset overeating. The body is better at protecting against starvation than against gluttony.

❚ FIGURE 7.2 The four components of energy output.

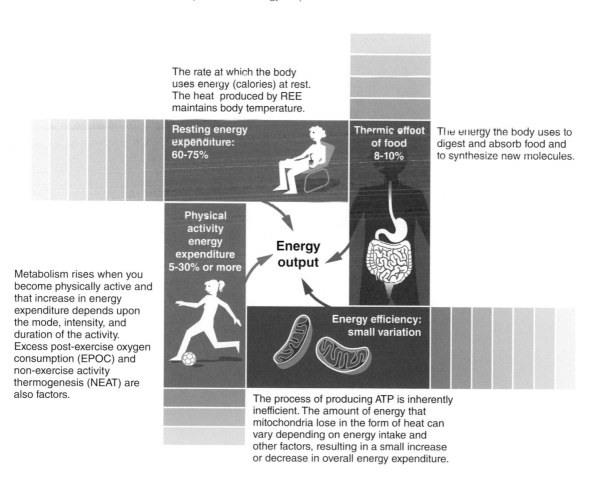

The rate at which the body uses energy (calories) at rest. The heat produced by REE maintains body temperature.

Resting energy expenditure: 60-75%

Thermic effect of food 8-10%

The energy the body uses to digest and absorb food and to synthesize new molecules.

Physical activity energy expenditure 5-30% or more

Energy output

Metabolism rises when you become physically active and that increase in energy expenditure depends upon the mode, intensity, and duration of the activity. Excess post-exercise oxygen consumption (EPOC) and non-exercise activity thermogenesis (NEAT) are also factors.

Energy efficiency: small variation

The process of producing ATP is inherently inefficient. The amount of energy that mitochondria lose in the form of heat can vary depending on energy intake and other factors, resulting in a small increase or decrease in overall energy expenditure.

As described in chapter 3, RMR varies with body size and composition, and is affected by eating habits, as discussed later in this chapter. The thermic effect of food (TEF) refers to the energy used in digesting and absorbing food and beverages. TEF is affected by the size and composition of meals and the body's hormonal response to those meals.

Energy efficiency is another factor that influences daily energy expenditure. As noted at the beginning of this chapter, the ATP-producing processes in cells are not 100% efficient, because a lot of the energy associated with metabolism and muscle contraction is lost as heat. Producing more heat and less ATP is inefficient because it increases fat and carbohydrate oxidation. That's bad for ATP production but good for weight loss.

> **Resting metabolic rate is the amount of energy the body uses at rest and can be further broken down by the organ systems using the energy. (See figure 7.3.)**

One interesting factor involving energy efficiency that has received attention recently is brown fat. Brown fat (brown adipose tissue) is commonly found in animals (especially hibernating animals such as bears). Brown fat cells have more than the usual number of mitochondria and capillaries of normal fat cells (white fat) and are inefficient in their production of ATP. The result is that brown fat breaks down a lot of fatty acids and produces a lot of heat, a handy advantage when you want to hibernate outdoors and you have enough body fat to last through the winter. Brown fat is also good for newborn babies. All humans are born with a small amount of brown fat (about 5% of body weight) to maintain body temperature after birth, because infants can't fend for themselves in that regard. As time goes by, people move more and develop the capacity to shiver (a great way to produce heat), and brown fat is no longer needed.

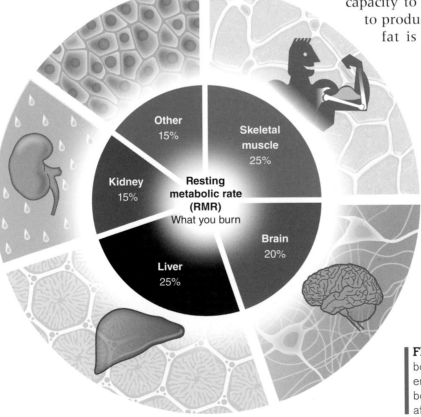

FIGURE 7.3 Resting metabolic rate (RMR) reflects the energy (calories) used by all body cells when the body is at rest.

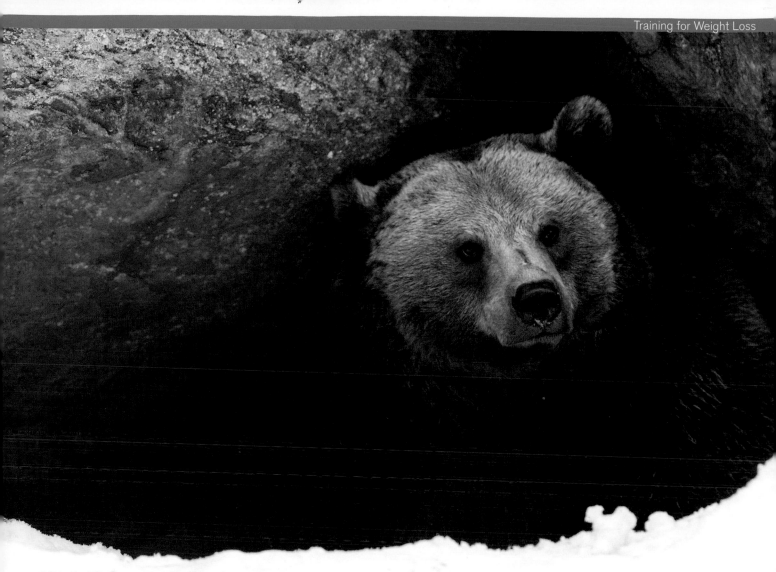

© Dieter Meyrl/iStock

However, some brown fat remains in adults and seems to increase in quantity as a result of prolonged exposure to cold weather. Beige fat cells appear to have characteristics between brown and white fat. This makes it theoretically possible that adults who have more brown or beige fat would have an easier time with weight control. You might have friends who seem to eat as much as they want and never gain weight. Could that be because they have more than their fair share of brown or beige fat? Brown and beige fat actually may be one reason some people have an easier time losing or maintaining weight than others. But, as in all things scientific, there are always other reasons.

The topic of brown and beige fat is interesting not only for its potential connection to weight control but also because it is an example of how regular physical activity stimulates a variety of responses that influence tissues throughout the body. Skeletal muscles, heart muscles, and fat all release hormones and other proteins into the bloodstream during exercise, perhaps as one way to communicate their needs to other tissues. For example, during exercise, heart and skeletal muscles release a hormone called irisin that appears to promote the transformation of some white fat cells into beige fat cells. This is just one example of how active muscle can communicate with the brain, liver, kidneys, bone, pancreas, and fat cells to produce short- and long-term responses that benefit overall fitness and health.

Physical activity energy expenditure is a large factor within

your control when it comes to weight management. The energy expended (Calories burned) during physical activity depends on many factors such as the type of physical activity, intensity of the activity, duration of the activity, and body weight. Table 7.1 contains examples of how energy expenditure varies among activities. Notice that continuous activities that involve many muscles, such as running and swimming, usually have a higher energy cost than intermittent activities, such as tennis. Of course, someone who swims leisurely will expend fewer Calories than someone playing an intense game of tennis, so the average values that you see in table 7.1 or find in other books or on the Internet are simply rough estimates of the average energy cost of activities.

The estimates of energy cost displayed on exercise equipment such as treadmills, stationary bikes, and elliptical trainers are just that—estimates. Those values are based on a variety of equations that differ from one piece of equipment to another. For example, you might input your age and body weight into a treadmill to allow it to estimate your energy expenditure based on those two variables plus the treadmill speed and elevation.

Regular exercise is the best single predictor of successful weight loss.

TABLE 7.1   **Average Energy Cost of Physical Activities Expressed in Calories per Minute (kcal/min) and Relative to Body Weight (kcal/kg/min)**

Activity	Estimated kcal/min (from MET values, assuming 1 MET = 1.5 kcal/min)	Relative to body mass (kcal/kg/min)
Basketball game	12.0	0.123
Cycling		
Cycling hard uphill	21.0	0.071
Cycling flat terrain (<10.0 mph)	6.0	0.107
Cycling flat terrain (>20 mph)	24.0	0.343
Running		
12.1 km/h (7.5 mph)	14.0	0.200
16.1 km/h (10.0 mph)	18.0	0.260
Sitting	1.5	0.024
Sleeping	1.0	0.017
Standing	1.8	0.026
Swimming laps, freestyle, hard	15.0	0.285
Tennis, singles	12.0	0.101
Walking, 3.2 km/h (2.0 mph)	3.0	0.071
Resistance training, vigorous	9.0	0.117

Note: Values presented are for a 70-kilogram (154 lb) person. These values will vary depending on many other factors and should be viewed as estimates that can give athletes and clients a sense of how energy expenditure varies among activities. The energy cost of other activities can be found at https://sites.google.com/site/compendiumofphysicalactivities/Activity-Categories.

Data from Ainsworth et al. Healthy Lifestyles Research Center, College of Nursing and Health Innovation, Arizona State University. https://sites.google.com/site/compendiumofphysicalactivities/Activity-Categories

It is impossible to determine just how accurate those estimates are regarding your actual energy expenditure because exercise equipment has no idea of how economically you are moving (reflected by your oxygen consumption at any given intensity), and you have no idea if the exercise equipment has been recently calibrated. So it's best to use that information only as general feedback.

Figure 7.4 depicts an interesting aspect of physical activity energy expenditure. *Nonexercise activity thermogenesis*, mercifully abbreviated as NEAT, is an interesting aspect of physical activity energy expenditure. NEAT can be thought of as accidental exercise because it encompasses the energy expended during daily activities such as standing, fidgeting, and stooping. You know people who just can't seem to sit still. Good for them, because fidgety people get a lot of accidental exercise; all those brief movements can add up to hundreds of Calories each day.

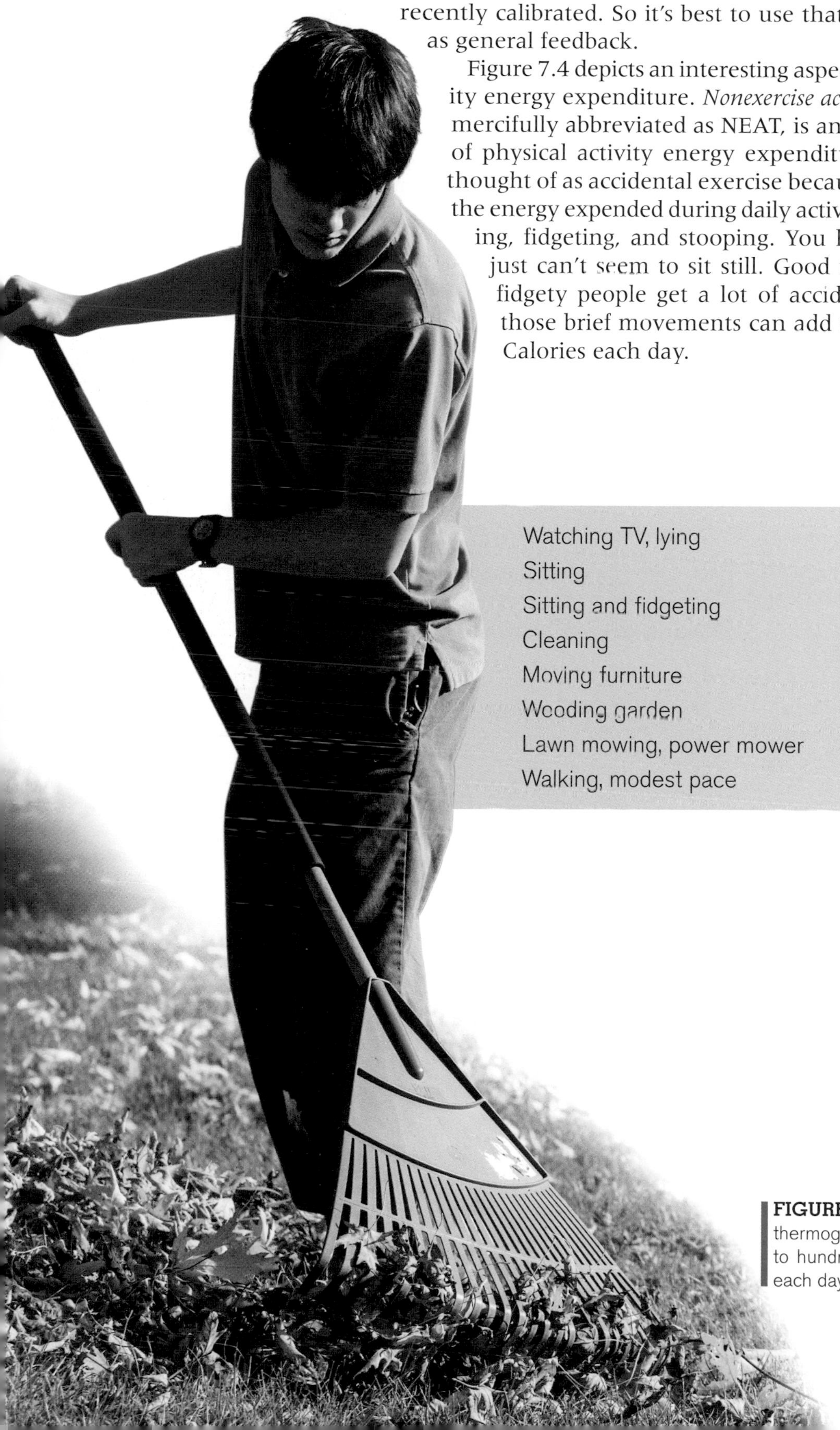

Watching TV, lying	1.0 kcal/min
Sitting	1.5 kcal/min
Sitting and fidgeting	2.0 kcal/min
Cleaning	3.0 kcal/min
Moving furniture	5.0 kcal/min
Weeding garden	4.0 kcal/min
Lawn mowing, power mower	5.0 kcal/min
Walking, modest pace	3.0 kcal/min

FIGURE 7.4 Nonexercise activity thermogenesis (NEAT) can amount to hundreds of Calories expended each day.

What's the Best Way to Estimate RMR?

To help athletes and clients understand their daily energy (Calorie) needs, it's helpful for them to understand their RMR. If you don't have access to equipment to measure oxygen consumption and lean body mass, then the next-best approach is to use equations to estimate RMR. Mobile phone apps and websites make the same estimates, so there's no need to belabor the topic here except to show that the equations look like those in table 7.2. To be most helpful, it makes sense to use more than one equation to create a range of RMR values that likely encompass the true RMR value for each person.

Measuring the resting metabolic rate (RMR) in a person who has severely restricted energy intake will underestimate true RMR because severe Calorie restriction causes the metabolism in many tissues to slow down.

Weight-Loss Supplements

Thousands of dietary supplements promise rapid weight loss. If that promise strikes you as too good to be true, that's because it is. Happily, this topic is a great example of the importance of the energy balance equation because the only way to lose fat weight is for energy intake to decrease or energy output to increase. For a dietary supplement to aid in fat loss would require the supplement to either reduce appetite (decrease energy intake) or increase resting metabolic rate (increase energy output). Is it possible for dietary supplements to do either? As you might imagine, a clear answer is hard to come by. Suffice it to say that the results of some studies of dietary supplements have shown small, short-lasting reductions in appetite and increased resting metabolic rate that are not much different in magnitude from the results brought about by placebo. This is true of a variety of herbal preparations and ingredients such as forskolin and garcinia cambogia as well as green tea extract and other caffeine derivatives. The dietary supplements that do reduce appetite are those that contain prohibited or dangerous substances such as prescription drugs or designer stimulants. Weight-loss supplements have been found to contain sibutramine (an amphetamine analog now banned for use in humans), fluoxetine (Prozac, an anti-anxiety drug), phenolphthalein (a chemical reagent), triamterine (a prescription diuretic), and even sildenafil (Viagra). Supplement contamination is a widespread problem because it is next to impossible for most people to decipher ingredient labels or keep up with the news about weight-loss supplements. To help in that regard, the U.S. Food and Drug Administration issues e-mail alerts to interested consumers whenever a supplement tests positive for a prohibited substance.

What's the Best Way to Estimate Daily Energy Needs?

The easiest way to estimate daily energy (caloric) needs is to multiply the estimate for RMR by a factor that roughly represents how active a person is on a daily basis. Again, it's most helpful for a client or athlete to create a range of daily caloric needs based on a high- and low-activity estimate. Table 7.3 has an example using the same volleyball player whose RMR was estimated in table 7.2. As with estimates of RMR, there are websites and phone apps that make similar calculations. Few people need the same amount of Calories day after day because daily energy needs vary depending on activity. Note in table 7.3 that there is a 1,000-Calorie difference in energy needs between the athlete's rest day and an intense training day.

TABLE 7.2 **Two Equations for Estimating RMR in Adults**

Equation	Men	Women	Example
Harris-Benedict	RMR (in kcal/day) = 66.473 + (13.7516 × body weight in kg) + (5.003 × height in cm) − (6.775 × age)	RMR (in kcal/day) = 665.0955 + (9.5634 × body weight in kg) + (1.8496 × height in cm) − (4.6756 × age)	20 year-old female volleyball player, 69 in. tall (175 cm), 136 lb (61.8 kg) RMR = 665.0955 + (9.5634 × 61.8) + (1.8496 × 175) − (4.6756 × 20) = 1,486 kcal/day
Mifflin-St. Jeor	RMR (in kcal/day) = (10 × body weight in kg) + (6.25 × height in cm) − (5 × age) + 5	RMR (in kcal/day) = (10 × body weight in kg) + (6.25 × height in cm) − (5 × age) − 161	20-year-old female volleyball player, 69 in. tall (175 cm), 136 lb (61.8 kg) RMR = (10 × 61.8) + (6.25 × 175) − (5 × 22) − 161 = 1,607 kcal/day

TABLE 7.3 **Estimating Daily Energy Needs From RMR and an Activity Factor**

Example: 20-year-old female volleyball player, 69 inches tall (175 cm), 136 pounds (61.8 kg)
Estimated average RMR = 1,546 kcal/day

Activity level	Activity factor	Energy needs
Rest day	RMR × 1.2	1,856 kcal
Light training day (e.g., ≤1 hr of light exercise)	RMR × 1.375	2,216 kcal
Moderate training day (e.g., 1 to 2 hr of moderate-intensity exercise)	RMR × 1.55	2,396 kcal
Heavy training day (e.g., 2+ hr of high-intensity exercise)	RMR × 1.725	2,667 kcal
Intense training day (e.g., 2+ hr of nonstop high-intensity exercise)	RMR × 1.9	2,937 kcal

Energy Balance Versus Energy Availability

Energy balance is the difference between energy input and energy output. When body weight does not change over time, energy balance is 0 Calorie per day because energy input minus energy output equals 0. If you eat too much, energy balance becomes positive and you gain weight. If you eat too little, energy balance becomes negative and you lose weight.

When energy input is restricted for prolonged periods (a few weeks or more of *energy deficiency*), RMR slows down as the body tries to compensate for reduced energy intake. When this happens, it becomes tougher to lose weight unless energy input continues to decrease. Athletes and fitness enthusiasts can experience energy deficiency as a result of *eating disorders* (e.g., anorexia nervosa), in misguided attempts to lose weight, unusual eating behaviors (often referred to as *disordered eating*, including fasting, laxatives, and induced vomiting), or because of an unintentional failure to eat enough.

Energy availability is a simple concept based on simple arithmetic: The difference between energy input and physical activity energy expenditure equals energy availability, the amount of energy that is available to meet the body's remaining needs for energy. Here is one example using the hypothetical female volleyball player. If she consumes 2,356 Calories on one day and expends 856 Calories during her training, her energy availability would be 2,356 − 856 = 1,500 Calories. For this particular day, the athlete would be in an energy deficit because her estimated energy needs in order to meet her RMR and basic daily activities (RMR × 1.2; see the calculations in table 7.3) is 1,856 Calories. If this pattern continued, the athlete would be in a state of energy deficiency and at risk for menstrual irregularities, loss of bone mineral content, and impaired performance in training and competition.

Calculating energy availability can be a tool in helping clients and athletes make informed decisions about strategies for weight loss and weight gain (see table 7.4). However, to have confidence in those calculations, you have to have an accurate idea of a person's typical daily energy input (in kcal/day), energy output (in kcal/day), body weight (in kg), and at least an approximation of fat-free mass (FFM, in kg). FFM is used in the following calculations to represent the energy needs of the most metabolically active tissues of the body.

TABLE 7.4 **Calculating Energy Availability to Recommend Strategies for Weight Loss and Gain**

Goal	Evaluate risk of energy deficiency	Safely lose weight	Maintain or gain weight
Calorie intake	<30 kcal/kg FFM/day	30-45 kcal/kg FFM/day	>45 kcal/kg FFM/day
Example	122 lb female high school cross-country runner consumes 2,200 kcal/day and expends 950 kcal/day in training. She wants to maintain her current weight but struggles during some training sessions and races.	192 lb 46-year-old male recreational basketball player consumes 3,460 kcal/day and expends 625 kcal/day in fitness training and basketball games. He wants to lose weight to improve his long-term health and increase his quickness on the court.	212 lb 16-year-old high school male football player wants to gain weight but has been having a difficult time doing so. He typically consumes 4,300 kcal/day and expends 1,200 kcal/day during weightlifting and team practice sessions.
Energy availability	2,200 − 950 = 1,150 kcal/day. She has 16.5% body fat, so her FFM = 122 − (122 × .165) = 102 lb (46.4 kg).	3,460 − 625 = 2,835 kcal/day. He has 22.3% body fat, so his FFM = 192 − (192 × .223) = 149 lb (67.8 kg).	4,300 − 1,200 = 3,100 kcal/day. He has 14.4% body fat, so his FFM = 212 − (212 × .14) = 182 lb (82.9 kg).
Lowest estimated energy availability	30 × 46.4 = 1,390 kcal to meet daily nonexercise needs. This value > current energy availability of 1,150 kcal/day.	30 × 67.8 = 2,034 kcal to meet daily nonexercise needs. This value < current energy availability of 2,835 kcal/day.	45 × 82.9 = 3,729 kcal to meet daily nonexercise needs. This value > current energy availability of 3,100 kcal/day.
Recommendation	She is at risk of performance and health consequences of energy deficiency. She should increase energy input or reduce training load so that energy availability exceeds 1,400 kcal/day.	He could reduce energy intake by no more than 500 kcal/day and safely lose weight without being in danger of energy deficiency.	He should increase energy intake by at least 650 kcal/day to begin to gain weight.

Why Do Some People Have Difficulty Losing Weight?

In one sense, losing weight can be as easy as moving more and eating less. For some people it *is* that easy. After all, the laws of thermodynamics can't be broken: If you ingest fewer Calories than you expend, you will lose weight over time. Yet for other people, moving more and eating less do not have the same satisfying results. In fact, some people who are on an identical regimen of exercise and diet don't lose much weight at all. Why is that? Some of the factors that affect weight loss are summarized in figure 7.5, and the following sections discuss in more detail some of the variation among individuals.

FIGURE 7.5 Many factors influence and complicate the energy balance equation regarding weight loss.

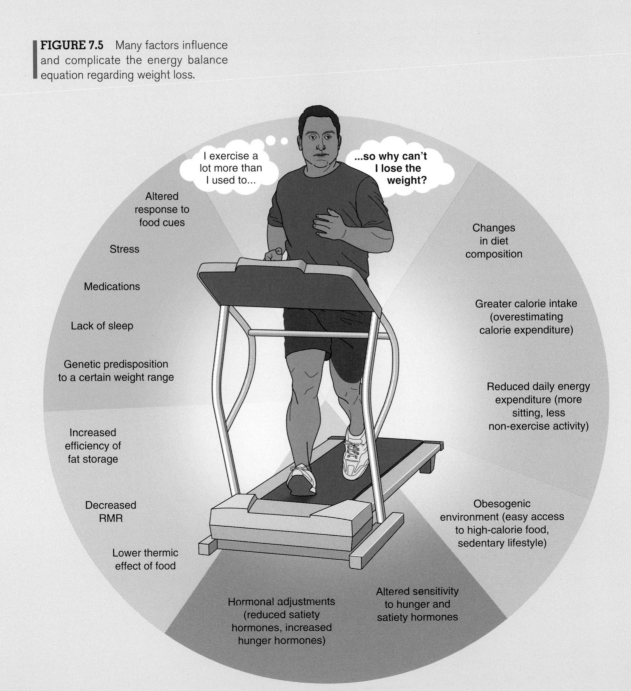

Genetics

You just can't seem to get away from your pesky genes. Some scientists think that genes determine body weight and make futile any attempt to establish a new body weight outside of a fairly narrow gene-determined range. Other scientists agree that genetics play a role in body weight but not as the sole determining factor. Otherwise, how do you explain people who lose hundreds of pounds and maintain their new lower weight for decades?

Homeostatic Compensation

This sounds more complicated than it is. The thinking is that the body has a set point for body weight, and attempts to alter weight provoke compensations to counter those attempts.

Here's a simple example: People who introduce exercise into their daily routine in an attempt to lose weight are often frustrated by the slow pace of weight loss. Research shows that when people begin to exercise regularly, they often increase their food intake and decrease their physical activity during the rest of the day. This also helps explain why people on very low-calorie diets often struggle to lose weight as the body tries to compensate for low energy intake by reducing RMR.

Consistently undereating decreases resting metabolic rate (RMR), the thermic effect of food (TEF), the energy cost of movement due to weight loss, nonexercise activity thermogenesis (NEAT; posture, fidgeting), and satiety hormones (e.g., leptin, insulin, cholecystokinin), while hunger hormones (e.g., neuropeptide Y, ghrelin) are increased. In other words, undereating results in compensatory metabolic and behavioral responses that combine to work against weight loss.

Hormones

The neuroendocrine system (brain, central nervous system, hormones) plays an important role in the regulation of hunger and satiety. Eating provokes the release of dozens if not hundreds of hormones from the brain, gut, pancreas, liver, and other organs, creating a rich mix of signals that influence feelings of hunger and satiety. Some people may be more sensitive to those signals than others, and that higher sensitivity means that hunger is turned off sooner, so they eat less and don't gain weight.

Undereating and overeating produce wide variations in weight loss and gain. For example, overeating 1,000 Calories per day results in storage of 100 to 700 Calories per day. Resistance to fat gain is explained by increases in NEAT, TEF, and energy expenditure.

What's the Best Way to Lose Fat but Protect Muscle Mass?

In chapter 6, you learned that muscle is very plastic; it adapts to the stress placed on it and even more quickly loses those adaptations when the stress is removed. Adding muscle mass requires the right type of exercise and the right type of diet with an emphasis on consuming enough energy (Calories) to increase or maintain muscle protein content. Along with adequate energy, muscles require carbohydrate, protein, and water for recovery, repair, and growth. Diets that restrict energy intake too severely run the risk of promoting muscle loss along with fat loss.

Clients and athletes who want to lose fat weight but maintain or increase muscle mass have to be careful about how much they restrict their energy intake. Large drops in energy intake (e.g., −1,000 kcal/day) will definitely result in weight loss, but some of that weight loss will be due to a loss in the size of muscle cells, because those cells break down contractile proteins to produce energy (ATP) and are unable to repair or replace damaged proteins. This loss of muscle can be reduced by increasing the amount of protein in the daily diet to 1.6 grams per kilogram (0.7 g/lb/day), twice the recommendation for protein intake in sedentary people. Very low caloric intake (e.g., 1,200 kcal/day or fewer) in adults provokes a compensatory decrease in RMR as the body tries to reduce its energy needs to cope with inadequate daily energy intake. Not surprisingly, a reduced RMR makes it much tougher to lose weight, one of the reasons experts recommend a sustained weight loss of 1 to 2 pounds per week as a result of moderate energy restriction (e.g., −250 to −500 kcal/day) and an increase in energy expenditure.

Smaller drops in energy intake (e.g., −250 to −500 kcal/day) result in slower rates of weight loss, but much less of the weight lost is muscle tissue. Even better responses occur when exercise is used to increase energy expenditure with little or no decrease in energy intake. For example, if a person needs 2,500 Calories per day to maintain current body weight, weight loss will occur if energy intake is reduced to 1,500 Calories per day. Weight loss will also occur and muscle mass will be better protected if the person increases energy output by 500 Calories per day or more along with establishing a modest decrease in energy input.

People who lose large amounts of weight have some things in common: Most eat breakfast every day. Most weigh themselves at least once each week. Most watch less than two hours of TV daily. And most exercise about an hour each day.

Aiming to lose fat weight at a gradual pace (i.e., 1 to 2 pounds, or 0.5 to 1 kg, of body weight per week) reduces the chance of regaining the weight and also reduces the impact on exercise and sport performance. This pace of weight loss minimizes the loss of both muscle and water. Losing weight at a more rapid pace means losing muscle mass and becoming dehydrated, two negative consequences that impair both health and performance. For athletes or people who are already active, maintaining or increasing physical activity energy expenditure while modestly reducing energy intake by 250 to 500 Calories per day is usually enough to promote a loss of 1 to 2 pounds of fat each week.

Compared to males at any relative BMI value, twice as many females perceive themselves as overweight. For example, a woman at the 50th percentile for BMI (i.e., 50% of women have a higher BMI and 50% have a lower BMI) is twice as likely as a man at the 50th percentile for BMI to feel overweight and to be engaged in trying to lose weight.

What's the Best Way to Lose Abdominal Fat?

This is one question that will always be asked, in large part because many people don't understand the basics of fat loss. The way in which fat is stored varies between sexes and among people. Many females deposit fat on their hips, leading to pear-shaped *gynoid obesity*. Many males tend to deposit fat in the abdominal region, leading to apple-shaped *android obesity*. Obviously not all women are shaped like pears, nor are all men shaped like apples. There is a wide range within the sexes in how fat is deposited throughout the body. That wide range also determines how fat is lost from the body. For example, a person who is genetically predisposed to accumulating fat in the abdominal area will first notice fat loss in that area, even though fat is being lost from fat cells throughout the person's whole body.

Loss of excess abdominal fat is the result of the loss of fatty acids from fat cells throughout the body, including the abdomen. Doing endless crunches and planks will strengthen the abdominal muscles and improve the chances that a six-pack will eventually emerge, but those exercises will not spot-reduce abdominal fat. Fat loss is enhanced by increasing energy output and reducing energy input. It's just impossible to stray far from the energy balance equation!

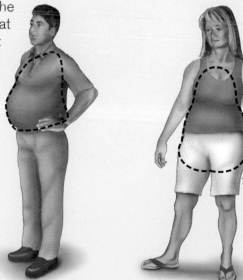

Upper body (android) obesity   Lower body (gynoid) obesity

Adapted, by permission, from W.L. Kenney, J.H. Wilmore, and D.L. Costill, 2015, *Physiology of sport and exercise,* 6th ed. (Champaign, IL: Human Kinetics), 562.

What Is the Fat-Burning Zone?

From a scientific standpoint, there is no one fat-burning zone. The body is constantly burning fat; the amount of fat being burned (oxidized to produce ATP) rises and falls depending on physical activity. The popular notion of the fat-burning zone is that there is a range of exercise intensity (often linked to exercise heart rate) that maximizes the amount of fat being burned during exercise. But as shown in figure 7.6, the total energy expended during exercise, not the source of that energy, is most important. Also note that the amount of fat oxidized *during* exercise is often very small; the total number of Calories expended during the day (total energy expenditure) determines how much fat is lost over time.

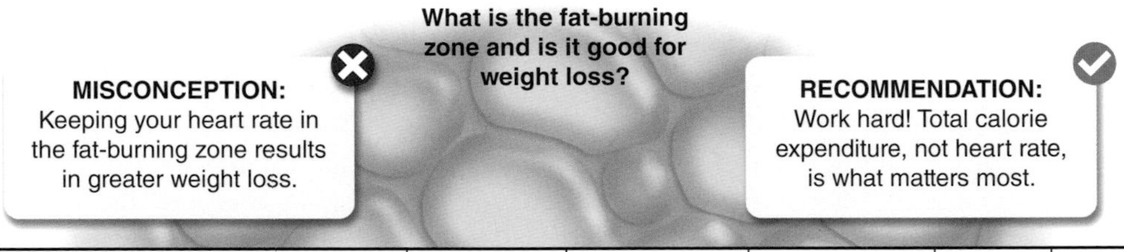

What is the fat-burning zone and is it good for weight loss?

MISCONCEPTION: ✗
Keeping your heart rate in the fat-burning zone results in greater weight loss.

RECOMMENDATION: ✓
Work hard! Total calorie expenditure, not heart rate, is what matters most.

		Intensity	$\dot{V}O_2$ (L/min)	% kcal from carbohydrate	% kcal from fat	kcal/hour
If you exercise at 50% of your maximal heart rate about 50% of ATP production will come from fat oxidation and 50% from glucose oxidation. 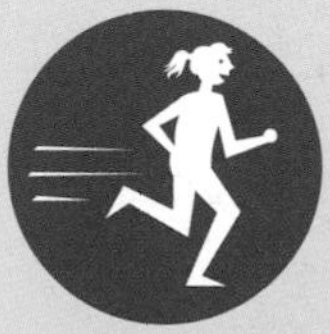		50% HR_{max}	1.50	50%	50%	440
Increase your intensity to 75% HR_{max}, and your fat oxidation will drop to 33% of ATP production. That drop might seem counterproductive to fat loss, but it isn't. Energy expenditure is greater at higher exercise intensities and that number is what counts in overall energy balance (or energy availability). 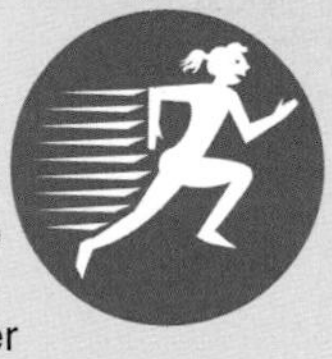		75% HR_{max}	2.25	67%	33%	664

In most cases, oxidation from fat stores during exercise = 1 oz/hour

FIGURE 7.6 The fat-burning zone is meaningless for weight loss because overall energy expenditure and energy intake are what determine fat loss over time.

Adapted, by permission, from W.L. Kenney, J.H. Wilmore, and D.L. Costill, 2015, *Physiology of sports and exercise*, 6th ed. (Champaign, IL: Human Kinetics), 568.

Does Consuming Calories During Exercise Defeat the Weight-Loss Purpose of Exercise?

Short answer: no. Look at figure 7.7 for an extreme example. It's easy to understand why people believe that if their goal is to lose weight, they shouldn't consume Calories during exercise—a time when they are working hard to expend Calories. Yet, research shows very clearly that ingesting carbohydrate Calories (energy) during a workout is associated with an increase in energy expenditure (more Calories burned) because the exercising muscles have an additional fuel source and can work harder. Keep in mind that overall energy expenditure during the day—the total of physical activity energy expenditure and nonexercise activity thermogenesis, or NEAT—determines total energy output.

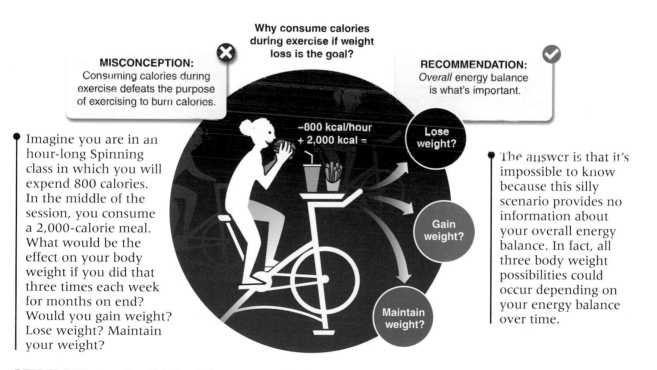

Why consume calories during exercise if weight loss is the goal?

MISCONCEPTION: Consuming calories during exercise defeats the purpose of exercising to burn calories.

RECOMMENDATION: *Overall* energy balance is what's important.

Imagine you are in an hour-long Spinning class in which you will expend 800 calories. In the middle of the session, you consume a 2,000-calorie meal. What would be the effect on your body weight if you did that three times each week for months on end? Would you gain weight? Lose weight? Maintain your weight?

−800 kcal/hour + 2,000 kcal =

Lose weight?

Gain weight?

Maintain weight?

The answer is that it's impossible to know because this silly scenario provides no information about your overall energy balance. In fact, all three body weight possibilities could occur depending on your energy balance over time.

FIGURE 7.7   Ingesting Calories during exercise in the form of sports drinks, carbohydrate gels, energy bars, or any other food source will not make it more difficult to lose fat. Weight loss depends on overall energy balance, not just the energy (Calories) consumed on a specific occasion.

Will Exercising While Fasting Increase Fat Oxidation and Weight Loss?

There is no doubt that fasting causes the body to limit its use of carbohydrate and rely more on the oxidation of fatty acids to produce ATP. So fasting does cause an increase in fat oxidation (fat burning). Similar increases in fat oxidation occur when consuming a high-fat diet. But as shown in figure 7.8, fasting reduces the body's use of carbohydrate during exercise and consequently its ability to maintain power output. That's not a good thing because reduced power also means reduced energy expenditure—fewer Calories are burned.

Although some people believe that high-fat diets are good for appetite control, fat is the weakest macronutrient at producing satiety and increasing its own oxidation. True high-fat diets deplete muscle and liver glycogen, leading to the loss of water molecules that are normally stored with glycogen. Water loss, not fat loss, explains most of the rapid weight loss that occurs in the early stages of such dieting.

Will training in a fasted state or when avoiding carbohydrates enhance muscles' ability to burn fat?

MISCONCEPTION:
Training fasted ramps up fat burning.

RECOMMENDATION:
It does, but performance suffers. You are likely to work out harder and burn more calories when carbohydrate stores are normal.

Fasting or low-carbohydrate, high-fat diets lead to

• Enhanced fat oxidation
• Impaired carbohydrate oxidation
• Lower workloads
• Altered immune response

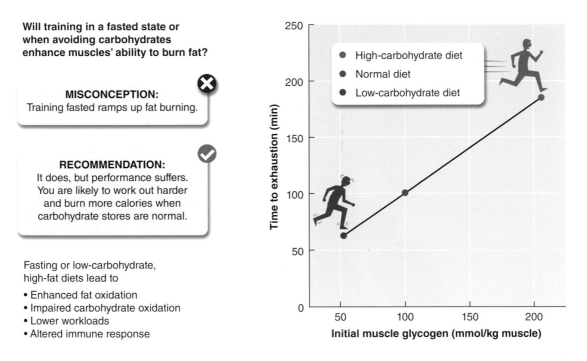

FIGURE 7.8 Fasting and low-carbohydrate diets do increase the amount of fat the body oxidizes (burns), but these practices also reduce the carbohydrate available to muscle (glycogen), which shortens the time to exhaustion and limits the ability to train at high levels.

Adapted, by permission, from W.L. Kenney, J.H. Wilmore, and D.L. Costill, 2015, *Physiology of sport and exercise*, 6th ed. (Champaign, IL: Human Kinetics), 382.

CHAPTER EIGHT

Training for Speed and Power

Proper training results in changes in muscles, connective tissues, and the nervous system that produce faster, more explosive athletes.

Speed and power are critical elements in all athletic events. Even for those uninterested in competition but desiring improved fitness, enhanced speed and power are unavoidable by-products of training. A football player tackling a ballcarrier, a wrestler shooting for a single-leg takedown, a volleyball player leaping for a spike, a gymnast executing a dismount, a swimmer exploding from the starting blocks, a basketball player sprinting the court to get back on defense, and a javelin athlete on the final step before a throw all exhibit a combination of speed and power. In those examples, it's easy to understand how improved speed and power are related to improved performance. But the same is true for a middle-aged woman newly enrolled in a fitness class, a recreational runner trying for a personal record in a 5K race, and a 74-year-old man working to regain leg strength after a hip replacement.

It's easy to understand why speed and power are important to athletes, and it's equally easy to understand why people interested in losing weight, improving muscle tone, or enhancing overall fitness would not think in terms of improving their speed and power as personal goals. Yet, all training programs influence speed and power, even when speed, power, and sport performance are of no interest to a client.

What Are Speed and Power?

Speed and power are inextricably linked because power is influenced by speed. You intuitively know what speed and power mean in the exercise and sport settings, but in a book like this one, it's good to begin with clear definitions of those terms. (See figure 8.1.)

Speed is a measure of the rate of motion; in math terms, speed (S) is the distance (D) traveled divided by the time (T) it takes to travel that distance:

$$S = D / T$$

When you can cover the same or more distance in less time, you've become faster. Your speed has increased.

Power is a measure of the rate at which energy is transferred; in sports, power (P) is force (F) multiplied by distance (D) and divided by time (T).

$$P = (F \times D) / T$$

In this simple equation, force (F) can refer to body weight or to the weight of a barbell or the resistance setting on a piece of exercise equipment. Power is determined by the amount of force and the speed at which that force is applied or resisted. For example, a football player becomes more powerful as he becomes faster, provided his body weight has not decreased. Increased power is particularly important in football, weightlifting, throwing sports, and sprint events of any kind. Speed and power usually improve together with training, but there are times when it makes sense to be more concerned with improving speed even if power decreases. That's certainly the case in all timed events in running, swimming, and cycling when finishing first is the goal. Generally speaking, power increases as a person becomes faster, but there are occasions when an athlete needs to lose fat weight to increase speed. If the decrease in body weight (F in the power equation) falls more than the increase in speed (D / T), then power will drop slightly, but that's of little consequence if the goal of increasing speed has been achieved.

Power is not often considered important for marathon runners and other endurance athletes, but both speed and power are critical for all sports. Speed in large part determines power, and the ability to generate greater amounts of power is just as important for endurance athletes as it is for football players and athletes in other explosive sports. Although endurance athletes generate far less maximal power than sprint athletes, endurance athletes are able to maintain power output for long periods. Sprinters and endurance athletes all must improve speed and power in order to improve their performance. Well-designed training programs improve speed, power, and endurance capacity.

Even with interval training and fitness classes of any sort, as people become more fit, lose weight, and improve their skills, their speed and power will be affected. While that improvement should not be the only goal for recreational exercisers, it's important to keep in mind that all types of training influence speed and power.

Speed is a measure of the rate of motion.
Power is a measure of the rate at which energy is transferred.

A 150-pound speedy halfback will not generate as much power when he hits the defensive line as will a slower 225-pound halfback. The heavier player has a slower rate of motion (speed) but a greater rate of energy transfer (power). If either athlete became faster, his power would increase. The same is true if either athlete gained muscle mass and maintained the same speed.

A volleyball player wants to be able to spike the ball more forcefully. Strength and skill training increase the muscle mass and strength in her shoulder and arm as well as the speed at which she hits the ball. Now the rate of her arm motion (speed) and the mass of her shoulder and arm have increased, resulting in a more powerful spike (increased rate of energy transfer).

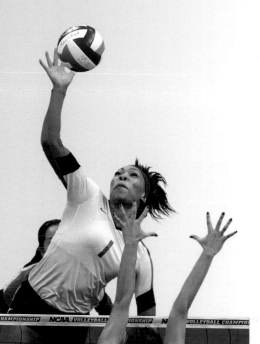

A 100-meter sprinter dedicates himself to off-season strength training in an attempt to become faster. His training is successful as he gains 12 pounds of muscle and gains strength in all his lifts, especially in his upper body. But his initial times are disappointing, significantly slower than at the start of the previous season. In this case, the increase in body mass slowed his rate of motion (speed), even though his rate of energy transfer (power) may have remained the same.

FIGURE 8.1 Speed and power are important factors in all athletic pursuits, from short sprints to ultra-marathons. The amount of power that the body generates during activity is related to speed of movement and the force (weight, also known as mass) being moved.

© technotr/iStock

What Adaptations Are Needed to Improve Speed and Power?

Increasing speed and power requires that active muscle cells be able to produce ATP at a higher rate, sustain that production rate for a longer time, and generate more force in the process. In this case, *force* refers to the strength of each contraction. Recruiting more motor units helps in achieving those goals, as does increasing the myofibril content of muscle cells. All of those adaptations are made possible by proper training.

Improving the capacity for exercise—any sort of exercise—requires the right stimulus (training) to provoke an optimal response (adaptation). Improvements in speed and power are no exception. Common sense combined with a little knowledge about training adaptations indicates that speed and power training should result in improvements in anaerobic ATP production along with increases in muscle strength and other changes needed to support a faster, more powerful athlete. Speed and power training results in a variety of adaptations that improve the capacity for high-intensity exercise.

Although speed and power training is of obvious importance for athletes in sports that require brief, explosive movements, because of the interconnectedness of the energy systems, aerobic training is also relevant for all athletes. You learned that ATP is constantly being produced from anaerobic (PCr and glycolysis) and from aerobic (Krebs cycle, electron transport chain) processes. This is true at rest and during all types of physical activity; muscle cells simply adjust their reliance on the energy systems based on how rapidly ATP must be produced. For example, even though the average American football play lasts only about 6 seconds, there is an endurance (aerobic) component to those brief, explosive activities, and the recovery periods that follow, especially when the players are on the field for extended periods.

Sport training always involves a combination of aerobic and anaerobic ATP production. Even shot putters require improved aerobic capacity to support their intense training sessions, even though during competition each effort lasts only a few seconds.

> An individual's genetics determines the upper limit of what training can accomplish, but no genes are linked strongly enough with performance to justify their use in predicting athletic success.

Benefits of Speed and Power Training

- Stronger muscles
- Bigger muscles
- Greater ATP production
- Faster ATP production
- Increased power
- Increased muscle fiber cross-sectional area
- Increased percentage of type II fibers
- Stronger connections between tendons and bones
- Stronger bones
- Faster reflexes
- Increased agility
- Improved skills at speed

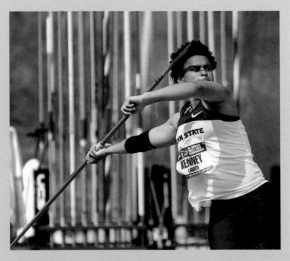

What Determines Competitive Success?

Why do some people excel at sports and others struggle? Look at any team in any sport and you'll find a range of fitness levels, sport skills, and competitive success, even though the team members are all exposed to similar training. So why is it that a similar stimulus results in various degrees of adaptation? The following figure provides some insight.

Health:
Injury and illness both play a major role in a person's capacity to adapt to training. Training programs are often derailed by injury and illness that limit the overall training stimulus. Adequate rest and sleep are also important aspects of maintaining good health.

Hydration:
Staying well hydrated during training and throughout the day supports important systemic functions such as a high cardiac output during exercise, but also positively impacts cellular functions. In short, a hydrated muscle cell favors anabolism (building up molecules), while a dehydrated cell favors catabolism (breaking down molecules).

Training:
Even genetically gifted, motivated athletes will struggle to find success if their training programs are not properly designed and implemented.

Adaptation:
Part of an athlete's genotype determines the extent of his or her adaptations to training. Some athletes adapt more quickly and to a greater extent than team members who are doing the same training. But adaptation is also impacted by the quality of the training program, including rest, recovery, nutrition, and hydration.

Nutrition:
Recovery from training and competition and the related intracellular and systemic adaptations are made possible by consuming the wide variety of macro- and micronutrients needed to provide fuel, repair cells, support growth, and stimulate adaptations.

Genetics:
A person's genotype establishes the upper limits for adaptation and improvement. Great athletes are born with a genotype that allows for large adaptations in response to the various stimuli of training.

Motivation:
While a person's genotype establishes the upper limit for what is possible with training, athletes who are motivated to succeed often find greater success because of their dedication and work ethic.

Supplements:
Compared to the major influence of other factors that affect athletic success, dietary supplements play a very small role, a role that is complicated by the fact that many supplements are ineffective and some supplements are contaminated with prohibited substances.

Many factors affect a person's success in sport. Some are within the athlete's control, and others are not.

What Kinds of Training Improve Speed and Power?

The *principle of specificity* (see chapter 5 for a refresher) indicates that adaptations to training are specific to the mode and intensity of the training. Common sense dictates that if you want to improve speed in the 100-meter sprint, it would be silly to train like an endurance athlete. Fortunately, a variety of approaches that can be integrated into any training program can enhance speed and power.

Interval Training

Interval training has been a staple of elite athletes since at least the 1930s. Interval training intersperses exercise and rest in an endless variety of ways and can be used with any sport or physical pursuit; programs can be designed for everyone, from sprinters to ultraendurance athletes. One advantage of interval training is that it allows for repeated high-intensity efforts that help maximize the exercise stimulus and optimize training adaptations. Interspersing bouts of exercise with rest periods allows for higher exercise intensities than what can be sustained during continuous exercise. High exercise intensity is a greater stimulus to provoke training adaptations because of the increased demands on the cardiorespiratory system, the metabolic systems required to produce ATP, the buffering systems needed to control acid buildup, the ability of the nervous system to recruit muscle motor units, and the capacity to store and use carbohydrate and fat, all of which result in the production of signals throughout the body.

The right combination of exercise intensity and rest (the work-to-rest ratio) depends on the athlete's fitness and training goals (figure 8.2). There is no single work-to-rest ratio that

Out-of-Shape Softball Player

Goal: Improve speed and agility. Reduce risk of knee injury.

The objective of this sample 45-minute interval training session is to practice proper running and jumping mechanics while completing exercises designed to improve quadriceps, hamstring, and core strength and stamina. As fitness and movement skills improve, the number of reps and sets can gradually increase and the rest intervals can decrease.

- Warm-up: 15-minute combination of walking, jogging, running, stretching.
- 3 sets of 30-yard jog, run, sprint, 1 every 30 seconds. Rest as needed.
- 4 reps of 30-second body planks: front, right, front, left, with 30-second rest between each.
- 4 reps of 10-yard agility squares: side shuffle right, backpedal, side shuffle left, sprint forward. One square every 30 seconds or rest as needed.
- 8 depth jumps, each from 1-foot height with soft, stable landing.
- 10 reps of stability-ball leg curls.
- Repeat 4 reps of 10-yard agility squares: side shuffle right, backpedal, side shuffle left, sprint forward. Rest as needed.
- Cool-down.

is optimal; the design of interval training workouts should reflect the objective of the training session and the overall goal of the training program. Here are some approaches to interval training:

- 30 seconds on and 30 seconds off for 12 minutes
- 4 reps of 3 minutes on and 3 minutes off
- 20 seconds all-out and 2 minutes off; repeat 6 times
- 12 × 100 yards every 90 seconds
- 6 stair sprints, 1 every 3 minutes

Circuit training is a form of interval training that usually involves a series of resistance and body-weight exercises (e.g., bench press, pull-up, biceps curl, leg extension, push-ups) with short rest intervals between each.

Completion of all the exercises represents a circuit. Fartlek training—also called speed-play training—was developed in Sweden in the late 1930s and is a hybrid of continuous training and interval training. In Fartlek training, continuous exercise at a sustainable intensity is periodically interrupted by bouts of high-intensity efforts typically lasting 30 seconds to 3 minutes. In recent years, research has shown that high-intensity interval training (abbreviated HIIT) is effective in improving aerobic and anaerobic fitness with minimal time commitment.

The *principle of specificity* is still a valid concept for sport training in that the bulk of training time should be devoted to sport-specific skill and fitness development. Until recently, the prevailing thinking was that endurance athletes should train primarily with long-duration

Collegiate Soccer Player

Goal: Improve end-of-game stamina and agility.

The objective of this sample 60-minute interval training session conducted in a fitness facility is to challenge the core and leg muscles before completing an agility drill and high-intensity sprints. Improved performances on the agility drill and high-intensity sprints at the end of the workout signal when to increase the reps and sets for the preceding exercises.

- Warm-up: 15 minutes on treadmill or cycle ergometer to break a sweat.
- 3 sets of 20 seated medicine-ball core twists, feet off the floor; 1 set every 45 seconds.
- 6 sets of 10 side planks with rotation, 1 set every 45 seconds, 3 sets each side.
- 3 sets of 8 deadlifts with barbells or dumbbells; 1-minute rest between sets.
- 3 sets of 20 side-to-side single-leg hops (10 on each leg); 1-minute rest between sets.
- 5 reps of slalom drill (10 small cones in a 5-yard line); sprint through, walk back. Record cumulative sprint time for future comparisons.
- 6 reps of all-out 20-second sprinting on a treadmill or cycle ergometer, every 2 minutes with light active recovery between each sprint. Record cumulative distance covered for future comparisons.

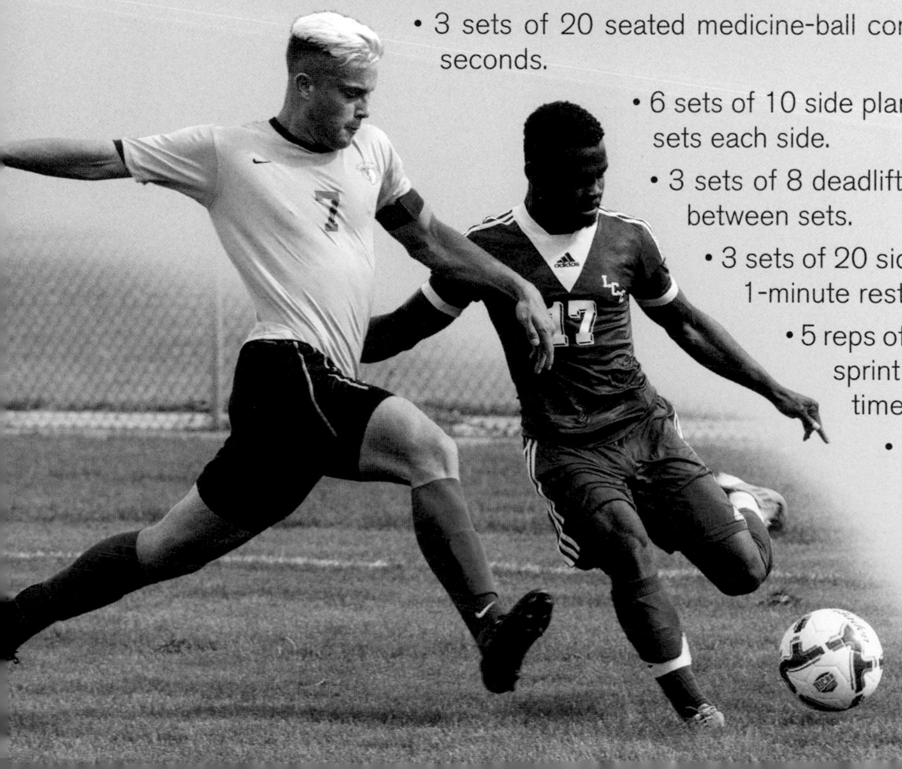

FIGURE 8.2 The appropriate work-to-rest ratio depends on the training goals.

bouts of exercise to mimic the demands of endurance sport. Although interval training has always been a staple of endurance training, very short-duration, high-intensity interval training was not considered an effective way to build endurance capacity. However, research has shown that some types of HIIT can benefit endurance performance. Research conducted on trained and untrained individuals shows that HIIT produces adaptations commonly linked with endurance training, such as increased concentrations of oxidative (aerobic) enzymes in muscle cells.[*]

[*]Gibala, M.J. 2007. High-intensity interval training: A time-efficient strategy for health promotion? *Current Sports Medicine Reports, 6*: 211-213.

HIIT Example

- 30-second all-out exercise
- 4-minute rest
- Repeat 5 times
- 3 sessions per week

Benefits

- Increased endurance capacity
- Increased muscle oxidative capacity
- Increased muscle glycogen
- Reduced lactate production

© Matt Brown/iStock

Determining Intensity for Anaerobic Training

Training intensity during workouts is typically monitored using heart rate, metabolic equivalents (METs), or rating of perceived exertion (RPE). A well-designed training program includes activities conducted at varying intensities, and only a small portion (e.g., 10-20%) of the weekly training load is conducted at very high intensity. As an athlete's or client's fitness improves, training intensity will naturally increase. Outside of a laboratory setting, monitoring training intensity is an imprecise science.

Heart rate is an obvious response to track during exercise because changes in heart rate are related to changes in oxygen consumption, the gold-standard measure of exercise intensity. Monitoring just heart rate is not very valuable unless you know the individual's maximum heart rate. Maximum heart rate can be measured during a progressive exercise test to exhaustion, or it can be estimated from equations developed in laboratory experiments. There are numerous formulas for estimating maximal heart rate (HR_{max}), the basis for establishing HR ranges (zones) that correspond to various exercise intensities.

Monitoring HR can be a gauge of exercise intensity, but it is important to keep in mind that HR is affected by dehydration, heat, illness, and other stresses that can cause misleading HR responses. For example, if an athlete is accustomed to training in a heart rate zone of 135 to 145 bpm (beats per minute) during endurance training, simply being dehydrated can increase heart rate, making it appear as though the athlete is working harder than she actually is. Dehydration requires the heart to beat faster to maintain cardiac output.

METs are often used in clinical settings such as cardiac rehabilitation and occupational therapy facilities to help monitor and control exercise intensity after heart surgery or injury. Exercise programs for older adults could incorporate the use of METs as a way to gauge progress in restoring or improving the physical capacity required for the tasks of everyday living.

Most people intuitively rely on some variation of RPE to adjust their exercise intensity to match the demands of exercise with how they are feeling during a workout or competition. Educating athletes and clients about the proper use of a simple RPE scale can be useful in establishing the intensity of effort suited to various tasks. Of course, RPE scales rely on the individual's assessment of and comfort with physical effort, so those differences among people introduce variability in their responses. As an example, if an instructor of a Spinning class asks the class to adjust the resistance on the bike to a "somewhat hard" level (e.g., RPE of 14 to 16 on a scale of 6 to 20), there will be a large variability among class members in the actual resistance settings on their bikes. Those who are diligent about their training will follow the instructions, while those who decide not to work as hard have that option. Motivated and experienced athletes and clients are accustomed to pushing themselves and adjusting their efforts to fit the demands of training and competition.

Research indicates that improving core stability and core strength does not appear to be linked to improved sport performance.

Plyometrics

Plyometric training is often a focus of athletes who want to increase power and speed. Stretching a muscle before it contracts adds to the force and power of the contraction. Virtually all human movements—especially sport movements—involve a combination of eccentric (lengthening) and concentric (shortening) contractions. Plyometric exercises such as box jumping and bounding help athletes take better advantage of stretch–shortening movements. The likely effects of plyometric training are described in figure 8.3.

Keep in mind that the eccentric contractions that are part of plyometric training increase the risk of muscle damage and injury, so athletes and clients should do such exercise sparingly and at low intensity until they become accustomed to the movements.

Eccentric training can enhance muscular strength and power by increasing muscle mass and the rate at which muscles develop force as well as increasing the length of muscle fasciculi and the number of sarcomeres in type II (fast-twitch) muscle fibers.

FIGURE 8.3 Plyometric training triggers several adaptations, including increased ability to generate power.

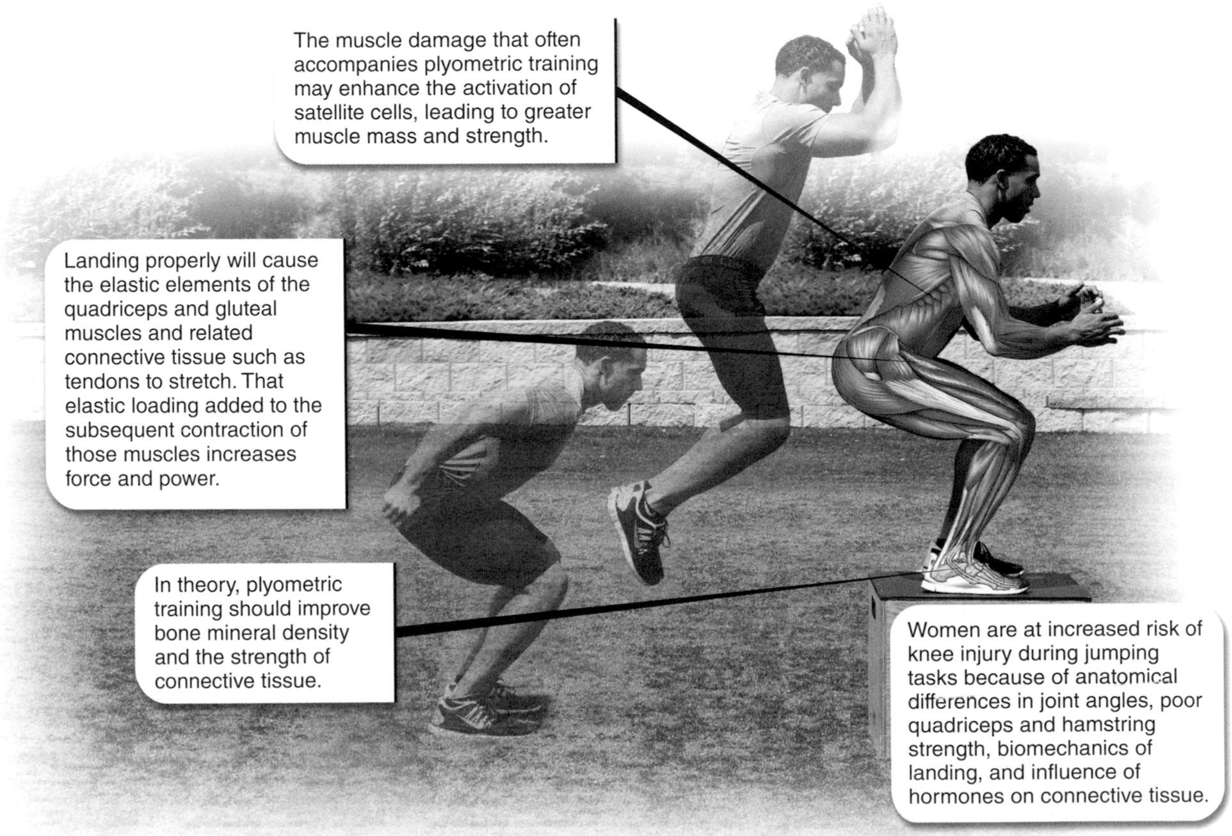

The muscle damage that often accompanies plyometric training may enhance the activation of satellite cells, leading to greater muscle mass and strength.

Landing properly will cause the elastic elements of the quadriceps and gluteal muscles and related connective tissue such as tendons to stretch. That elastic loading added to the subsequent contraction of those muscles increases force and power.

In theory, plyometric training should improve bone mineral density and the strength of connective tissue.

Women are at increased risk of knee injury during jumping tasks because of anatomical differences in joint angles, poor quadriceps and hamstring strength, biomechanics of landing, and influence of hormones on connective tissue.

Cross-Training

Cross-training provides variety to workouts. It also develops complementary new skills and promotes training adaptations that might otherwise be missed in sport-specific training. There appears to be little risk in cross-training provided it does not detract from time spent developing sport-specific skills and fitness. An example of cross-training is a triathlete who has to train in swimming, cycling, and running, often combined with strength training and flexibility exercises. Other examples of cross-training include wrestlers and swimmers who run and cycle, football and basketball players who participate in aerobic dance classes, and ice hockey players who circuit train. Proper cross-training should introduce mental and physical variety and complement the overall intent of the training program. Proper cross-training has to have a well-defined purpose. It makes no sense for basketball players to participate in aerobic dance unless the anticipated outcomes are clearly defined ahead of time and match the training needs of the athletes. Here are a few things to keep in mind when planning how to integrate cross-training into an athlete's training schedule:

- Endurance benefits are not blunted by appropriate strength training. In other words, strength training can be part of an endurance athlete's training program without concern that it will interfere with endurance-related adaptations.

- Strength benefits can be blunted by too much endurance training. Research indicates that strength development can be blunted somewhat by concurrent endurance training, something to keep in mind when designing training programs for individuals for whom strength development is the primary training objective. As an example, an athlete who has had a leg immobilized for weeks because of injury will have lost muscle mass and strength. Introduc-

ing endurance training too soon in the return-to-play training program will risk blunting strength development.

- Cross-training can result in improvements in endurance, strength, and power that are complementary to sport performance.

- Cross-training can also help reduce the risk of overtraining and overuse injuries in susceptible athletes or as part of a return-to-play training plan after injury.

Combining resistance training with endurance training may produce an interference effect that limits gains in muscle mass, strength, and power because endurance training stimulates intracellular signals that limit muscle contractile protein synthesis.

What Does a Speed and Power Training Session Look Like?

Table 8.1 provides an example of a speed and power training session. As with all types of training sessions, there are endless ways to mix the elements of speed and power training to create variety and maximize the training stimulus.

Improvements in performance of vertical jump occur with a combination of plyometric and resistance training.

TABLE 8.1 **Sample 30-Minute Speed and Power Training Session**

Phase	Goals	Exercise	Time or reps
Warm-up	Increase heart rate, breathing, core temperature in preparation for harder efforts	Jump rope	2 min
Plyo box *Circuit format × 2; 20-sec recovery between sets *From a plyo box or stand; explosive but controlled movements	Intersperse explosive eccentric movements with sprinting to improve speed and power	Jump-up	8 reps
		Sprint	1 all-out sprint of 20 to 60 yd
		Depth jump	8 reps
		Sprint	1 all-out sprint of 20 to 60 yd
		Lateral push-off	8 reps
		Sprint	1 all-out sprint of 20 to 60 yd
Med ball Circuit format × 2; 20-second recovery between sets	Intersperse core, throwing, and eccentric movements with sprinting to improve speed and power	Kneeling twisting throw	8 reps
		Sprint	1 all-out sprint of 20 to 60 yd
		Broad-jump throw	8 reps
		Sprint	1 all-out sprint of 20 to 60 yd
		Supine power drop	8 reps
		Sprint	1 all-out sprint of 20 to 60 yd
Barbell Alternate exercises	Improve lower-body strength and stamina	Squat with bar in front	6 reps × 3, 20 sec recovery between sets
		Calf raise	15 reps × 3, 90 sec rest between sets
Dumbbell Alternate exercises	Improve upper-body strength and stamina	Shoulder press	6 reps × 3, 20 sec recovery between sets
		Lat pullover	15 reps × 3, 90 sec rest between sets

Sample workout by Kelly Schnell, BS, CSCS, ACSM-CPT.

Dietary Supplements for Speed and Power

Hundreds of sport supplements claim they can improve speed and power, but few of those claims are supported by competent science. Nothing beats the right combination of proper training and nutrition to support the adaptations to training. The right sport supplement might provide a small additional performance benefit but only if a solid foundation of proper training and food-first nutrition is already in place.

Some supplements have been shown to be associated with improved speed and power output, at least in laboratory settings. Creatine and beta-alanine are two examples of dietary supplements that have been shown to increase speed and power. Creatine supplementation has been shown to improve repeated high-intensity exercise performance, so creatine loading could be a performance aid in training sessions that include repeated explosive movements. Beta-alanine is an amino acid supplement that may increase the ability of muscle cells to buffer lactic acid, helping to sustain high-intensity efforts.

Before recommending a supplement to an athlete or client, you need to consider the risk-to-benefit relationship of supplement use. Is there a demonstrated benefit? If so, what are the related risks to health or competition eligibility due to the possibility of banned substances? These are not easy questions, and it is always best to seek the advice of someone qualified to sort through the science and provide advice. Sport dietitians (registered dietitians—RDs—with training in sport nutrition) are trained to assess the risk-to-benefit ratio associated with the use of dietary supplements.

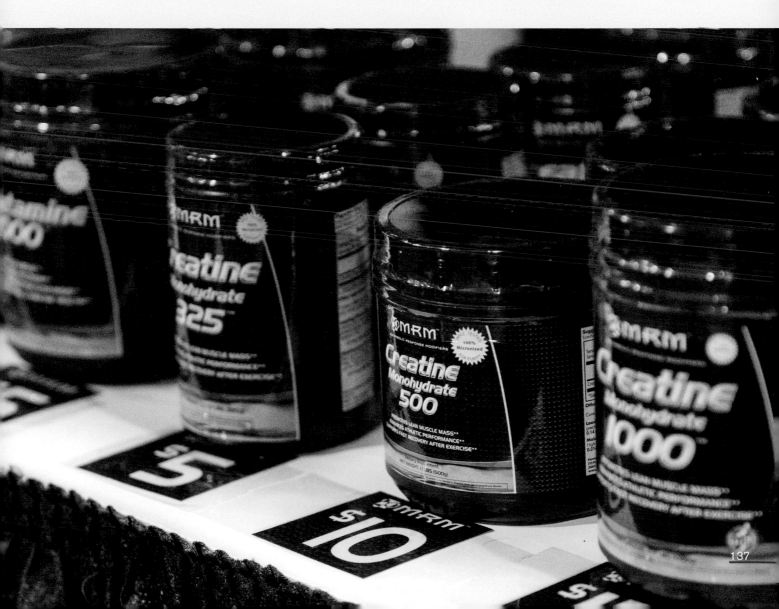

CHAPTER NINE

Training for Aerobic Endurance

The ability to exercise longer and harder requires the body to adapt to a combination of aerobic and anaerobic training.

When you think of aerobic endurance, it's natural to think of marathon running, cross-country skiing, road cycling, open-water swimming, and other sports and activities of long duration. After all, success in those kinds of activities requires a large aerobic capacity; in other words, success in endurance events requires a large $\dot{V}O_{2max}$, among other characteristics. But aerobic capacity is just as important in everyday life. Although many top endurance athletes have $\dot{V}O_{2max}$ values in excess of 70 ml/kg/min (60 ml/kg/min in women), at the other end of the spectrum are individuals for whom a $\dot{V}O_{2max}$ of just 15 ml/kg/min is needed to accomplish the basic tasks of everyday living. In contrast, young sedentary men and women have $\dot{V}O_{2max}$ values of 30 to 40 ml/kg/min. Proper training can obviously increase $\dot{V}O_{2max}$, and the extent of that increase depends on a variety of factors, only some of which are under an athlete's or client's control.

What Are the Main Adaptations to Aerobic Training?

Muscles use oxygen to produce much of the ATP required for contracting muscle cells and fueling other tissues throughout the body. At rest, you breathe slowly but at a rate sufficient to expose the lungs to ample oxygen and flush out the carbon dioxide resulting from energy metabolism. Oxygen molecules enter the bloodstream, bind to hemoglobin molecules in red blood cells, and are transported through arteries, arterioles, and capillaries for delivery to individual cells. Once inside cells, the oxygen molecules enter the mitochondria for use in the electron transport chain for the continuous production of ATP. During exercise, all those events accelerate: Breathing rate and depth increase, the heart beats faster, the left ventricle fills with more blood, cardiac output increases, arterioles dilate, and more capillaries fill with blood. Inside muscle cells, the increased oxygen delivery is matched by increases in the rate of glycogen breakdown, fatty-acid catabolism, glycolysis, lactate production, the Krebs cycle, and the electron transport chain. All of those events are reflected by one measurement: $\dot{V}O_{2max}$. The higher the $\dot{V}O_{2max}$, the faster the muscles can produce the ATP required for contraction.

An increase in $\dot{V}O_{2max}$ is one of many adaptations that occur with endurance training. Because it is one of many adaptations, a high $\dot{V}O_{2max}$ is not necessarily a good predictor of successful endurance performance. For example, there is no doubt that a person with a $\dot{V}O_{2max}$ of 55 ml/kg/min has a competitive advantage over someone with a $\dot{V}O_{2max}$ of 40 ml/kg/min, but the advantage may not hold true when competing against someone with a $\dot{V}O_{2max}$ of 50 ml/kg/min. In essence, $\dot{V}O_{2max}$ is simply a measure of the body's ability to extract oxygen from inhaled air and deliver it into the mitochondria in active muscle cells. There is an upper limit to that ability, and that upper limit is in large part determined by the heart's capacity to pump blood, the cardiac output. The upper limit for cardiac output determines the capacity not only for endurance exercise but also for the ability to

Mitochondria contain more than 1,000 different proteins. Training increases the number of mitochondria, antioxidants within mitochondria, and a variety of proteins that protect the muscle cells against stress.

live independently later in life. Not all people aspire to be endurance athletes, but all people do value the freedom associated with being able to take care of themselves. People engage in training to enhance functional capacity, be it to improve physical performance or simply to improve quality of life.

The most important adaptation for athletes is improved performance. Better performance is also an interest of exercise scientists because improving the capacity for exercise is important not only for athletes but also for everyone because improved aerobic fitness is related to a reduced risk of noncommunicable diseases such as heart disease, obesity, and diabetes; improved recovery from surgery; and all the other health-related issues listed in figure 9.1.

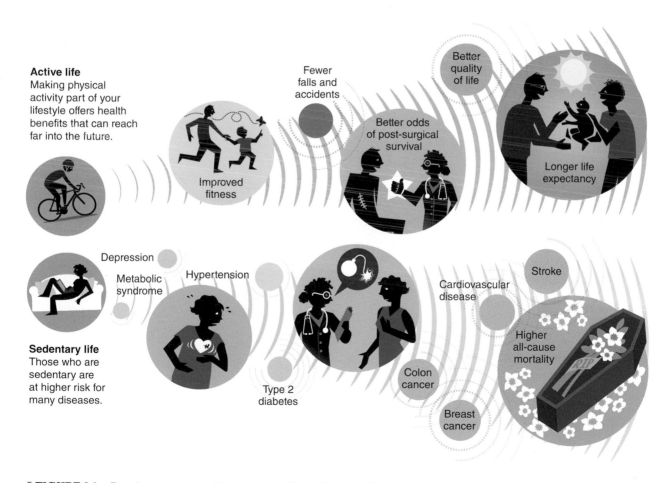

Active life
Making physical activity part of your lifestyle offers health benefits that can reach far into the future.

Improved fitness

Fewer falls and accidents

Better odds of post-surgical survival

Better quality of life

Longer life expectancy

Sedentary life
Those who are sedentary are at higher risk for many diseases.

Depression

Metabolic syndrome

Hypertension

Type 2 diabetes

Cardiovascular disease

Stroke

Colon cancer

Breast cancer

Higher all-cause mortality

FIGURE 9.1 Regular exercise and the improved fitness that results help reduce the risk of many diseases and disorders.

Why Is $\dot{V}O_{2max}$ So Important for Endurance?

Aerobic capacity—as measured by $\dot{V}O_{2max}$—reflects the capacity of muscles to produce ATP from the aerobic metabolism of carbohydrate (glucose) and fat (fatty acids). To improve fitness and endurance performance, the ability to produce ATP aerobically has to increase. That ability is reflected in $\dot{V}O_{2max}$. The higher the $\dot{V}O_{2max}$, the greater the ability to produce—and continue to produce—ATP.

As mentioned, the athlete with the highest $\dot{V}O_{2max}$ does not always finish first. Many other factors interact to determine overall athletic success; in endurance sports, $\dot{V}O_{2max}$ is just one of those factors. However, it is one of the major factors in the ability to complete endurance events.

Athletes and clients who want to improve their endurance have to complete the right amount and type of training in order to reach their performance goals. Figure 9.2 summarizes the main physiological changes that underlie an improvement in $\dot{V}O_{2max}$. Training programs—including nutrition, hydration, and rest—should improve all of these responses.

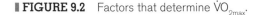

▮ FIGURE 9.2 Factors that determine $\dot{V}O_{2max}$.

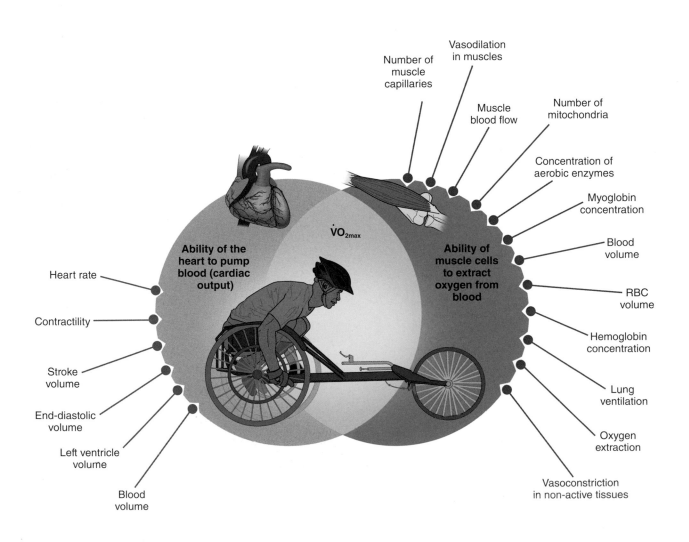

What Factors Determine How Much Aerobic Capacity Improves?

An obvious answer to this question is training. Adhering to an endurance training program is perhaps the single most important factor that determines how much aerobic capacity ($\dot{V}O_{2max}$) improves. However, individual response to an aerobic training program can vary. Following are key factors that combine to determine the overall improvement in $\dot{V}O_{2max}$:

- **Initial fitness.** An athlete with a high $\dot{V}O_{2max}$ before training will have a smaller improvement than an athlete who begins training with a low $\dot{V}O_{2max}$.

- **Heredity.** Genes establish the upper limit of improvement in $\dot{V}O_{2max}$ as the result of training.

  - **Sex.** $\dot{V}O_{2max}$ in women is typically 10% to 15% lower than that in similarly trained men.

  - **High or low responder.** Genetics (heredity) also determines the extent to which people respond to training. High responders improve quickly and to a greater extent than low responders.

    - **Training.** Even after $\dot{V}O_{2max}$ plateaus with training, endurance performance can still improve in terms of movement economy and anaerobic threshold.

In a muscle, mitochondria are located beneath the sarcolemma and between the myofibrils. These two types of mitochondria seem to differ in how they respond to training.

What Role Does Ethnicity Play in Endurance Performance?

Ever since the late 1960s, East African runners—from countries such as Ethiopia and Kenya—have been consistently successful in middle- and long-distance running events. Does their heredity—their genetic makeup—give those runners a competitive advantage that other racers cannot hope to achieve? Or do nongenetic factors such as living at altitude or being very active as children interact to produce supremacy in distance running? This puzzle has not yet been solved, but the following are key characteristics that likely combine to help explain the success of East African distance runners.

Heredity:	a genetic predisposition for a high aerobic capacity
Physically active as kids:	extensive running and walking throughout childhood
Living and training at altitude:	stimulate high hemoglobin, hematocrit, and blood volume
Body size and dimensions:	longer legs and a shorter torso favor better running economy
Muscle fiber type:	a higher percentage of type I fibers with great oxidative capacity
Traditional diet:	help speed recovery and promote adaptations to training
Economic motivation:	success at distance running is seen as one way to improve economic and social standing

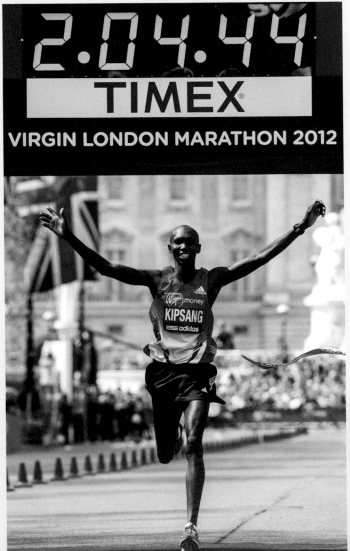

Wilson Kipsang Kiprotich is an elite Kenyan distance runner who has won the London, New York, Berlin, and many other marathons, as well as an Olympic bronze medal in the marathon. He is the former world record holder for this distance (2:03:23).

Why Is the Anaerobic (Lactate) Threshold Important?

As lactic acid (lactate) builds up inside muscle cells during intense exercise, some of it spills into the bloodstream, raising the level of blood lactate. During endurance exercise, blood lactate levels increase from resting values and then remain fairly steady until the push for the finish line. If exercise intensity creeps too high, blood lactate begins to accumulate, indicating that the active muscle cells are relying more and more on glycolysis —anaerobic metabolism—to produce ATP. If exercise intensity is not reduced, it becomes tougher to maintain the increased pace; before too long, fatigue sets in and the pace is forced to slow.

Proper training can increase the anaerobic threshold and reduce the accumulation of lactate. That means a faster pace of exercise, even if $\dot{V}O_{2max}$ remains unchanged (see figure 9.3).

● An athlete who can increase his anaerobic threshold from 75% to 88% of $\dot{V}O_{2max}$ can also increase the running speed he is able to maintain even if $\dot{V}O_{2max}$ remains unchanged.

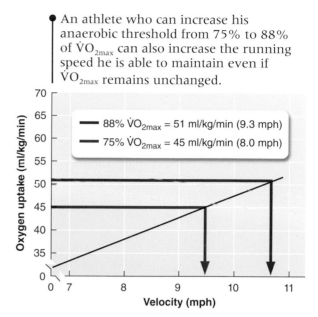

88% $\dot{V}O_{2max}$ = 51 ml/kg/min (9.3 mph)

75% $\dot{V}O_{2max}$ = 45 ml/kg/min (8.0 mph)

FIGURE 9.3 Improved anaerobic threshold increases race speed even without an increase in $\dot{V}O_{2max}$. This simple graph shows how an improvement in anaerobic threshold from 75% to 85% of $\dot{V}O_{2max}$ translates into a much faster sustainable race speed.

Based on W.L. Kenney, J.H. Wilmore, and D.L. Costill, 2015, *Physiology of sport and exercise*, 6th ed. (Champaign, IL: Human Kinetics), 265.

Lactic acid is a fuel that heart and skeletal muscles can use to benefit performance.

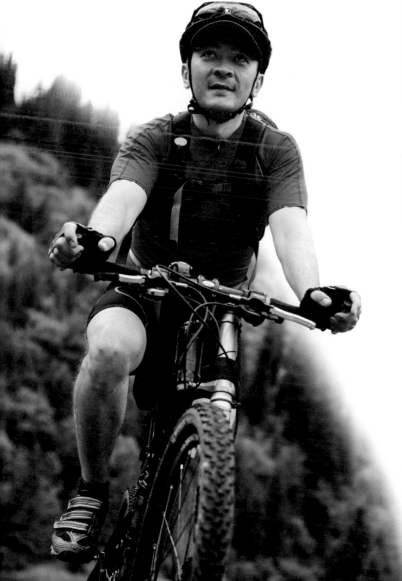

What Other Factors Affect Endurance Performance?

Remember not to confuse aerobic capacity and endurance performance. Although the two are definitely linked—those with greater aerobic capacities tend to have better endurance performance—aerobic capacity eventually plateaus with training, yet endurance performance can continue to improve for years.

One important characteristic in all sports is the energy cost of locomotion, which is referred to as *economy of movement*. Economy of movement is critical for endurance sports because uneconomical movements require ATP energy that does not contribute to forward motion. A simple example of the importance of movement economy is excessive bouncing while running. Each bounce requires energy that is not used for forward progress. Some of that lost energy with each bounce is elastic energy, not ATP energy, but it's also important for athletes to capture the elastic energy in muscles and connective tissues to contribute to forward movement.

Figure 9.4 shows the factors that sport scientists believe are determinants of endurance performance. Training programs for endurance athletes should reflect these characteristics.

> Some sport scientists think that in ultraendurance activities such as 100-mile runs, running economy is not as important as other factors—such as lactate threshold—in determining performance.

∎ FIGURE 9.4 Determinants of endurance performance.

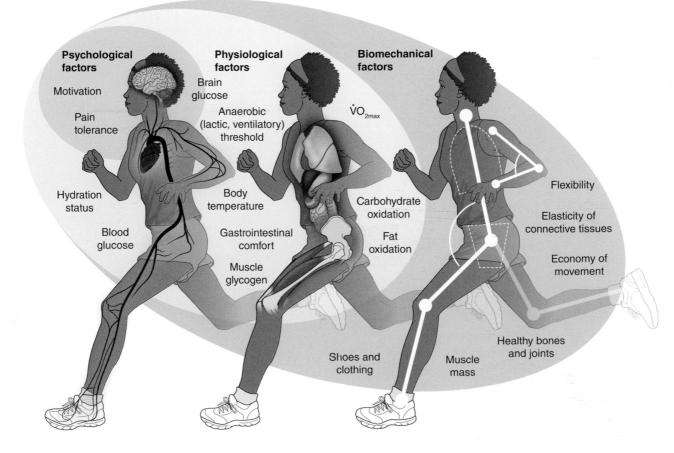

Psychological factors
- Motivation
- Pain tolerance
- Hydration status
- Blood glucose

Physiological factors
- Brain glucose
- Anaerobic (lactic, ventilatory) threshold
- Body temperature
- Gastrointestinal comfort
- Muscle glycogen
- $\dot{V}O_{2max}$
- Carbohydrate oxidation
- Fat oxidation
- Shoes and clothing
- Muscle mass

Biomechanical factors
- Flexibility
- Elasticity of connective tissues
- Economy of movement
- Healthy bones and joints

What Is Hematocrit and Why Should I Care About It?

Hematocrit is the scientific name referring to the percentage of blood that is composed of red blood cells. Determining a person's hematocrit is a simple procedure but is best conducted in a laboratory by someone trained and experienced in measuring hematocrit. A small amount of blood is drawn into a thin glass tube and then the tube is spun in a centrifuge to separate the blood cells from the plasma. Simply measuring the length of the total portion composed of the red blood cells and comparing that to the length of the entire content of the tube provide the hematocrit as a percentage of the total.

As with everything in biology, there is no one value that represents normal. In men, hematocrit is usually about 45%; in other words, 45% of the blood volume is taken up by red blood cells. In women, the average value is around 40% when normally hydrated. Dehydration artificially increases hematocrit because it reduces plasma volume.

Blood doping and injections of *erythropoietin* (EPO) have been used by some endurance athletes to increase the number of red blood cells, raising the hematocrit and the oxygen-carrying capacity of blood to boost performance. Some athletes do have naturally high hematocrit levels, but most people have lower levels. (Normal ranges are 41% to 50% for males and 36% to 44% for females.)

Some people mistakenly believe that hematocrit level increases after months of training as the body produces more RBCs as an adaptation to training. As shown in the illustration, the normal response is for hematocrit to fall slightly with training because even though the body does produce more RBCs, the increase in plasma volume (the fluid part of the blood) is greater than the increase in RBCs. The blood still carries and delivers more oxygen because there are more RBCs and a greater blood volume.

Hematocrit levels in excess of 50% increase the risk of heart problems, blood clots, and strokes because blood viscosity rises with hematocrit, making it harder for the heart to pump blood and more likely for clots to occur.

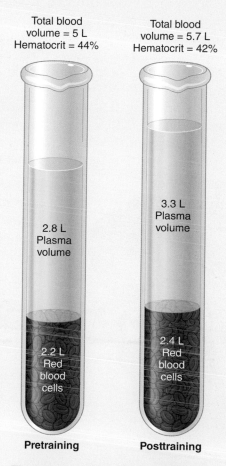

Total blood volume = 5 L
Hematocrit = 44%

Total blood volume = 5.7 L
Hematocrit = 42%

2.8 L Plasma volume

3.3 L Plasma volume

2.2 L Red blood cells

2.4 L Red blood cells

Pretraining

Posttraining

Though training increases both the number of blood cells and the overall blood volume, posttraining hematocrit is actually lower because the plasma volume increases more than the number of blood cells.

Reprinted, by permission, from W.L. Kenney, J.H. Wilmore, and D.L. Costill, 2015, *Physiology of sport and exercise*, 6th ed. (Champaign, IL: Human Kinetics), 271.

What's the Best Way to Improve Aerobic Endurance?

There is no one best way to improve endurance performance. Endurance athletes across sports have achieved great success using a variety of training approaches. Perhaps the best guidance is that training has to be suited to the physical and psychological characteristics of the athlete and adjusted to where the athlete lives; an endurance athlete who lives in a large city will train differently than if she lived in a hilly rural area. Success is achievable in both scenarios, but the training approach will be different.

Endurance athletes have achieved international and Olympic success by relying on interval training of varying distances, including repeats of 100-meter runs. Long slow distance training (LSD) has worked for many, as has threshold training designed to improve the anaerobic threshold. Hill training, fartlek training (speed-play training incorporating increased pace at different intervals during a long-duration effort), high-intensity interval training, strength training, and flexibility exercises can all be part of successful endurance training. The same holds true for those uninterested in sport but motivated to improve fitness; all of the same training approaches can be used during low-intensity walking, swimming, biking, and other activities.

Increasing cardiac output, elevating anaerobic threshold, and improving the economy of effort should be the top goals of training programs for endurance athletes.

When designing a training program to improve aerobic capacity and endurance performance, here are some general guidelines that can be manipulated to suit training programs of varying durations and goals:

❶ **Start out light and fun**—whether for an experienced athlete returning from the off-season or for someone new to training. The objective is to develop a solid training base as the foundation for the longer, more demanding training to come. Here are examples:

- Strength training circuit with light weights and high reps that gradually progresses over weeks to heavier weights and fewer reps.

- Low-intensity, low-mileage walks, runs, rides, and swims focusing on proper mechanics (improved economy of movement), with the occasional hill or similar challenge to begin building stamina. Gradually increase duration and distance over weeks. Less focus is on increased intensity.

- No more than twice each week, a short session of interval training that acquaints the athlete or client with the demands of high-intensity interval training. Gradually increase intensity over weeks.

❷ **Gear up for more**—preparing for competition. Once a satisfactory training base has been established and the competitive season is approaching, athletes should be physically prepared and mentally motivated to step up training intensity and duration. For clients interested in improved fitness, this phase of training will get them to the next level.

- Emphasis of strength training switches to developing sustained muscular power along with the improved core strength required for endurance competition. This is also a time to introduce simple agility exercises that endurance athletes often neglect as well as focus on exercises that develop sport-specific strength.

- Gradually increase the duration and intensity of training, incorporating a mix of anaerobic threshold training, low-intensity and long-duration efforts, speed-play (fartlek) training, and high-intensity interval training (HIIT).

- Increases in training intensity and duration should be gradual, with built-in periods when training load plateaus or even decreases for a few days to allow for recovery and adaptation.

- Continue to emphasize the importance of proper mechanics.

❸ **Training during the competitive season. Once competitions begin**—or in the case of the fitness client, once a new level of fitness has been established—the training program should change to reflect the added stress of competition as well as the need for continued improvement while reducing the risk of injury and overtraining.

- Strength training transitions from weight and machine resistance training to body-weight exercises and resistance bands to maintain or improve strength gains, with a continued emphasis on sport-specific movements.

- The duration and distance of long efforts now level off and the intensity gradually increases to reflect the demands of the competitive events.

- High-intensity training is limited to one day per week; other sessions are devoted to low-intensity recovery training and sessions with limited durations of sustained race-pace training.

❹ **Tapering for championships.** This period of the training season can differ dramatically depending on the nature of the championship event and the individual needs of the athletes or clients. Tapering should begin from 2 to 4 weeks ahead of the final event, customized to the individual's physical and psychological needs for reduced training and rest.

- Strength training transitions into a maintenance and injury-prevention program using stability balls and body-weight exercises.

- Endurance training backs off in overall intensity but maintains aspects of duration and distance that reflect the championship events. Limited threshold training helps sustain the speed required for racing.

Endurance training suggestions courtesy of Bill Bishop at Bishop Racing (www.bishop-racing.com).

If the benefits of training are specific to the type of training, then the majority of an endurance athlete's training should include activities that stress the aerobic production of ATP from carbohydrate and fat. With that obvious observation in mind, why should endurance athletes spend any time doing anaerobic training? Your common sense has probably already provided an important part of that answer: Endurance athletes need some sprint capacity—some anaerobic capacity—to pass competitors quickly and to sprint to the finish line when needed. But, as this list illustrates, there are other ways endurance athletes can benefit from high-intensity anaerobic training.

In short, high-intensity anaerobic training benefits endurance athletes by helping to maintain sprint capacity and providing an additional stimulus for producing the adaptations required for improving aerobic capacity.

Other variations of high-intensity training can benefit aerobic capacity and performance. Lactate threshold, anaerobic capacity, and even aerobic capacity can be improved by training that integrates repeated high-intensity bouts in an endurance workout. As an example, exercising hard for 3 minutes and then easier for 5 minutes, repeated throughout an hour-long run, cycle, or cross-country ski workout, can improve anaerobic threshold. Endless variations of this kind of speed-play (fartlek) training as well as classic interval training can add variety and high-intensity challenge to endurance workouts.

Benefits and Characteristics of High-Intensity Anaerobic Training

- High-intensity interval training increases both aerobic and anaerobic ATP production in muscle cells.
- Repeated sprints or high-intensity exercise bouts lasting 20 seconds to 3 minutes, followed by low-intensity activity, improve anaerobic and aerobic capacity.
- High-intensity interval training can be accomplished in as little as 20 minutes.
- A small amount of high-intensity interval training is as effective as a much larger amount of traditional endurance training at improving endurance performance.
- High-intensity anaerobic training should not totally replace conventional aerobic training, but it can be used periodically to give endurance athletes a new challenge that will benefit their performance.

Should Endurance Athletes Engage in Strength Training?

This topic is covered briefly in chapter 8, and it's good news for endurance athletes. The short story is that the benefits of endurance training are not reduced by strength training (but the benefits of strength training can be blunted by too much endurance training). A well-designed strength training program can help endurance athletes maintain or even build muscle mass, an important adaptation during long training seasons.

Although endurance runners and cyclists are often lean, maintaining adequate muscle mass is important for sustaining performance. Loss of muscle mass due to heavy training and inadequate energy (caloric) intake will impair performance. A 30-minute strength training program conducted twice each week can be enough to help prevent the loss of muscle mass.

Open-water swimmers, triathletes, cyclists, and cross-country skiers are good examples of endurance athletes for whom upper- and lower-body musculature is important for success in their sports. Off-season and in-season strength training is essential for increasing strength and preserving or enhancing muscle mass, adaptations that allow endurance athletes to train and compete at higher levels.

As an example, if a distance swimmer's maximal strength in the latissimus dorsi before a competitive season is 100 pounds and each race requires the swimmer to exert 65 pounds with each arm stroke, the swimmer is repeatedly using 65% of maximal strength. If that swimmer were able to increase maximal strength in the latissimus dorsi to 120 pounds, swimming at the same pace would require only 54% of maximal strength, making the effort easier. If the swimmer picked up the pace to use 65% of new maximal strength, the applied force would be 78 pounds, enabling the swimmer to go faster at the same relative effort as before.

Why Is Endurance Capacity Important for Sprinters and Team-Sport Athletes?

Increased aerobic capacity is the primary defense against fatigue for any athlete or client regardless of sport or activity. Even high-intensity sports stress athletes' aerobic capacity because recovery from repeated explosive movements relies on aerobic metabolism. And low-intensity sports such as golf and baseball have an important aerobic component because of the long duration of those activities.

Fatigue can hinder performance in all sports. Improved aerobic capacity can delay the onset of fatigue, benefitting performance even in nonendurance sports. Such activities don't rely on aerobic ATP production during competition, but the ability to continue to sustain mental concentration, recover from repeated explosive bouts of exercise, and withstand the heat all benefit from improved aerobic capacity.

That does not mean that a baseball player needs to train like a cross-country runner. But it does mean that a baseball player can benefit from training designed to improve his aerobic capacity. That type of training will not be a large portion of the player's overall training regimen but should not be neglected.

Effects of Fatigue on Performance

- Reduced power
- Impaired concentration and alertness
- Impaired agility and coordination
- Reduced strength
- Reduced speed
- Slower reaction and movement times
- Increased risk of injury

PART III

Special Considerations

CHAPTER TEN

Heat, Cold, and Altitude

Training and competing in different environments can present special challenges that make it tougher for the body to perform at its peak.

Heat, cold, and altitude are environmental stressors that affect the physiological responses to exercise, altering the body's ability to maintain speed and power. In simple terms, performance in cool weather is usually better than in cold or hot weather; performance at altitude in many events is impaired but in some events can be enhanced (e.g., sprinting, jumping, and some throwing events).

In this chapter, environmental stressors are tackled one at a time because that's a good way to illustrate how the body adjusts and adapts in commonsense ways to various environments.

Exercise in the Heat Impairs Performance

And it doesn't even have to be hot for performance to suffer. Research demonstrates that temperatures over 60 °F (15.5 °C) are hot enough to impair performance during prolonged exercise, compared to exercising in temperatures of 40 to 60 °F (4.4-15.5 °C). As the temperature rises above 60 °F, the negative effect on performance becomes greater. Exercising in the heat places an enormous stress on the cardiovascular system; not only is the heart required to pump a lot of blood to active muscles, but it also has to pump a lot of blood to the skin so that heat can be lost to the environment. In addition, the brain is very sensitive to heat, so whenever internal (core) temperature rises too high, the brain tries to slow down the body—and heat production—to prevent core temperature from rising too high.

Figure 10.1 illustrates the fundamental aspects of heat production and loss (heat balance) during exercise. The heat produced by muscles during exercise has to be lost to the environment to prevent rapid overheating. During vigorous exercise, most heat is lost by the *evaporation of sweat* from the skin. On cool days or in cool rooms, you also lose heat by *radiation* as heat moves from your warm body to the cooler surroundings. You can also lose additional heat with the help of *convection*, as you do on windy days or by exercising in front of a fan. *Conduction* is the final avenue for heat loss or gain, but it requires direct contact between the body and a cooler or warmer object. A hockey player lying on an ice rink is one example of conductive heat loss.

Dehydration and hyperthermia are closely linked because dehydration reduces the heart's ability to supply active muscles with blood or supply skin with enough blood to aid in heat loss. Staying hydrated during exercise helps protect blood volume and the heart's ability to deliver blood to muscles and skin.

Humans are homeotherms: Core temperature is regulated within a narrow range at rest (36.1-37.8 °C, 97.0-100.0 °F).

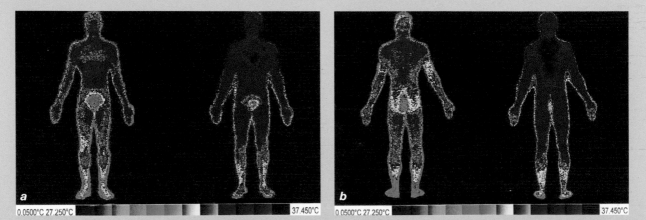

Infrared images showing the heat leaving the (a) front and (b) rear surfaces of the body before and after a run outside in hot, humid weather. In each pair, the pre-run image is shown on the left and the post-run image, on the right.

From Department of Health and Human Performance, Auburn University, Alabama. Courtesy of John Eric Smith, Joe Molloy, and David D. Pascoe. By permission of David Pascoe.

From a practical standpoint, for the best performance during hard workouts and competitions, it is always better to be cooler than warmer. Warm-ups should accomplish just that—warm up the muscles but keep internal temperature from rising too high. Some athletes use cold vests and cold-water immersion, rest in air-conditioned spaces, or consume cold drinks or ice slushies to lower body temperature in advance of all-out efforts because research shows that performance in the heat is improved by precooling.

Environmental heat stress cannot be measured by temperature alone. Environmental heat stress is determined by wind speed, humidity, radiation, and temperature.

FIGURE 10.1 Body temperature naturally rises during exercise as muscles produce heat that must be lost to the environment to keep internal temperature from climbing dangerously high. Depending on the environmental conditions, heat gain and loss can occur through various channels.

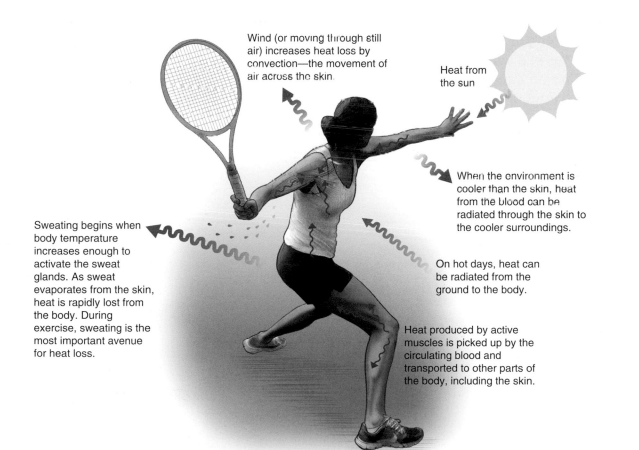

Wind (or moving through still air) increases heat loss by convection—the movement of air across the skin.

Heat from the sun

When the environment is cooler than the skin, heat from the blood can be radiated through the skin to the cooler surroundings.

On hot days, heat can be radiated from the ground to the body.

Sweating begins when body temperature increases enough to activate the sweat glands. As sweat evaporates from the skin, heat is rapidly lost from the body. During exercise, sweating is the most important avenue for heat loss.

Heat produced by active muscles is picked up by the circulating blood and transported to other parts of the body, including the skin.

Training in the Heat Improves Performance in the Heat

How can it be that exercising in the heat impairs performance but training in the heat improves performance? Performance in hot environments is consistently worse than in cooler environments because the body has only so much blood to go around. When blood flow to the skin rises to high levels, as it does during heat exposure, blood flow to muscles cannot rise high enough to sustain peak performance. But training in the heat—becoming *acclimated* to the heat—improves performance in all environments because of the many adaptations that accompany heat acclimation. Those adaptations are shown in figure 10.2 and are why many elite athletes undergo heat-acclimation training to improve all-weather performance.

Full heat acclimation requires training in a warm environment. Just being exposed to heat at rest is not enough.

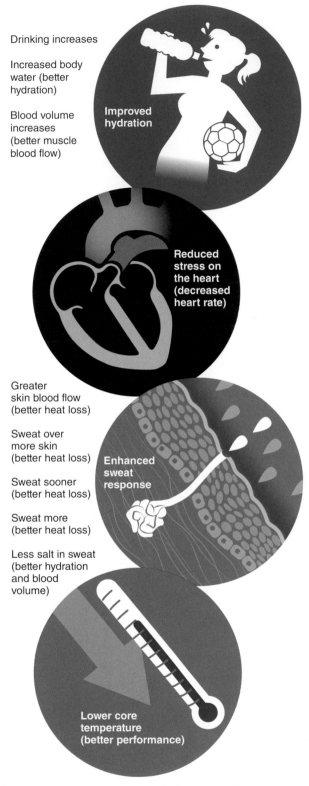

Drinking increases

Increased body water (better hydration)

Blood volume increases (better muscle blood flow)

Improved hydration

Reduced stress on the heart (decreased heart rate)

Greater skin blood flow (better heat loss)

Sweat over more skin (better heat loss)

Sweat sooner (better heat loss)

Sweat more (better heat loss)

Less salt in sweat (better hydration and blood volume)

Enhanced sweat response

Lower core temperature (better performance)

FIGURE 10.2 Acclimation to the heat occurs by training in warm weather. Gradually increasing the duration and intensity of workouts over the first two weeks of warm-weather training causes the body to undergo a variety of adaptations that improve the capacity to exercise in the heat.

Sweat Is Cool

You know what it's like to sweat, but few understand the true importance of sweating during physical activity or heat exposure. Whenever core body temperature rises above the *sweat threshold*, sweat glands in the skin begin to produce sweat. You were born with roughly two million sweat glands that enable you to survive hot weather and vigorous physical exercise simply because those glands secrete water onto the surface of the skin. As water molecules evaporate from the skin, heat is lost to the environment. In fact, during intense exercise, 80% of the heat produced by muscles is lost to surroundings by the evaporation of sweat. Sweat that drips off the skin, however, provides no cooling.

Sweating does for humans what panting does for dogs, but sweating does it better. Sweating is an effective way to stay safely cool in hot environments. That simple fact explains why humans are better than most animals at being physically active in the heat for prolonged periods. Animals that do not sweat cannot pant fast enough to keep up with the heat production of exercise. In humans, when body temperature increases slightly above normal resting temperature (98.6 °F, or 37 °C), the hypothalamus in the brain senses the increase in temperature and signals the sympathetic nervous system to dilate blood vessels in the skin and activate sweat glands. (See figure 10.3.)

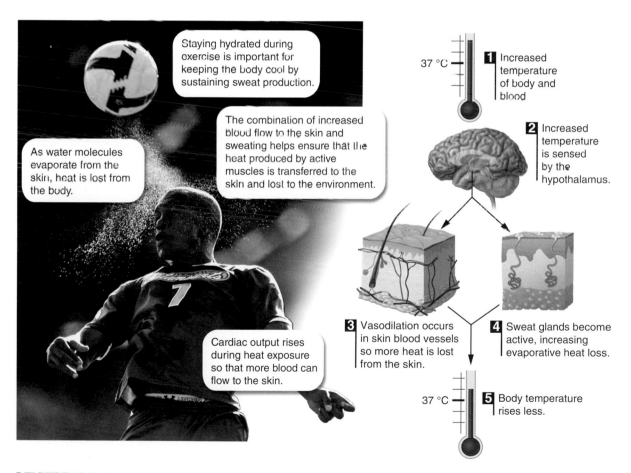

FIGURE 10.3 Sweating is a critical part of temperature regulation because sweating during exercise is the primary way in which humans lose heat to the environment and maintain a safe internal body temperature.

You know how uncomfortable you feel on a hot, humid day. The relative humidity of the air influences the rate of heat loss because humidity affects the evaporation of sweat. When the air is completely saturated with water vapor (100% humidity), sweat cannot evaporate from the skin; it literally has no place to go because the surrounding air already contains as much water vapor as it can hold. At the other end of the humidity spectrum, when exercise takes place in a dry, desert environment, sweat can evaporate so quickly from the skin that you hardly notice you're sweating. That rapid evaporation makes for effective heat loss but increases the risk of dehydration because sweaty skin and clothing are a cue that you're losing fluid and should drink to replace it. As humidity climbs above 50%, heat loss is made progressively more difficult, increasing the risk of heat exhaustion and heatstroke.

Dangers of Exercise in the Heat

There is a limit to the body's ability to lose heat to the environment. When that limit is reached, core temperature will continue to climb if exercise continues. The brain can tolerate internal temperatures of 40 to 41 °C (104-106 °F) for only short periods. The rate at which core temperature increases depends on the intensity and duration of exercise and the environmental conditions. Intense exercise in a hot, humid environment can cause core temperature to quickly climb to dangerous levels. In fact, if heat loss is impeded, body temperature can increase into the danger zone in just 15 to 20 minutes at a running pace of 10 minutes per mile. If core temperature remains at that high level for even a few minutes, *heatstroke* can result. Heatstroke is often fatal because being too hot for too long impairs brain function and causes proteins throughout the body to unravel. The result can be organ system failure and death.

Heat cramps and heat exhaustion are other forms of heat illness but are not life threatening. *Heat cramps* can result from the combina-

Individual sweating rates during the same activity vary widely from person to person, ranging from as little as 300 milliliters (10 oz) per hour (10 oz/hr) to over 3,000 milliliters (100 oz) per hour.

tion of intense exercise and dehydration. In some athletes, large sodium losses in sweat can cause severe, whole-body muscle cramps. *Heat exhaustion* occurs when dehydration reduces cardiac output and creates feelings of unusual fatigue and lightheadedness. Resting in a cool area and consuming cold beverages are usually all that are required to correct heat cramps and heat exhaustion.

Athletes have died from heatstroke in part because they exercised too hard for too long in hot environments. In addition to understanding heat balance during exercise, keeping athletes safe during hot-weather exercise requires that recognition of the main risk factors associated with heat illness.

Factors That Increase the Risk of Heat Illness

- Exercise intensity
- Air temperature
- High humidily
- Wind speed
- Heat sources in addition to the sun (e.g., overhead lighting, radiators, hot tubs)
- Dehydration
- Clothing and equipment that interfere with heat loss
- Being out of shape
- Being unaccustomed to the heat
- Being sick
- Being hungover

Heatstroke is often accompanied by collapse, confusion, and sometimes unconsciousness and is a medical emergency that must be dealt with quickly. Other symptoms of heatstroke include a core temperature of over 104 °F (40 °C), increased heart rate, decreased blood pressure, and rapid breathing. While emergency help is on the way, the athlete's torso should be submerged in an ice-water bath to quickly reduce core temperature. If an ice bath is not available, continuous cooling with cold water and wet towels can be used. Doing so saves lives.

Hot Yoga: Help or Hype?

Hot yoga (Bikram yoga) is a form of yoga exercise consisting of 26 yoga postures during 90-minute sessions in an environment maintained at approximately 104 °F (40 °C) and 40% relative humidity. Truly a hot and sweaty environment. What benefits can be expected from hot yoga? Answering that question requires some reading to identify the benefits that are claimed for hot yoga and the evidence in support of those claims.

The official Bikram yoga website notes that "these 26 postures systematically work every part of the body, to give all the internal organs, all the veins, all the ligaments, and all the muscles everything they need to maintain optimum health and maximum function. . . . Yoga changes the construction of the body from the inside out, from bones to skin and from fingertips to toes. So before you change it, you have to heat it up to soften it, because a warm body is a flexible body. Then you can reshape the body any way you want. . . . When you sweat, impurities are flushed out of the body through the skin."

There is not a lot of scientific research on hot yoga, although a few studies have been conducted. The results of the research confirm what you might expect: Yoga exercise is associated with a modest increase in oxygen consumption ($\dot{V}O_2$) and therefore energy expenditure. Novice yoga students tend to expend less energy than experienced students—a range of approximately 200 to 500 Calories per 90-minute session. That amounts to roughly 2 to 6 Calories per minute, qualifying as light to moderate exercise.

Not surprisingly, practicing yoga in the heat raises core temperature and heart rate and provokes sweating. In fact, one study noted that heart rates averaged 72% to 86% of HR_{max}, and novice students had lower values. Heat stress under any circumstance increases strain on the cardiovascular system because of the increase in blood flow to the skin and the loss of body water through sweat. Preventing dehydration by drinking adequate volumes of fluid is essential for protecting cardiovascular health and keeping core temperature from rising to dangerous levels. In addition, exposure to hot environments is contraindicated for those who have multiple sclerosis or cardiovascular disease.

Although there is no reliable evidence that exercise in the heat "softens" the body or that sweat flushes out toxins or impurities, practitioners of hot yoga will experience the physiological benefits of heat acclimation along with the modest improvements in strength, flexibility, and aerobic fitness associated with light to moderate exercise.

Pate, J.L., & Buono, M.J. (2014). The physiological responses to Bikram yoga in novice and experienced practitioners. *Alternative Therapies in Health and Medicine, 20*(4):12-18.

Bikram's Yoga College of India. (2015). Bikram yoga. www.bikramyoga.com/BikramYoga/about_bikram_yoga.php.

Cold Stress Chills Performance

Many environmental conditions can cause the body to lose heat rapidly and reduce core temperature. Fortunately, physical activity produces heat; although cold-weather sports such as ice hockey, downhill skiing, cross-country skiing, and football often take place in frigid conditions, the athletes remain warm provided their clothing restricts some heat loss. Figure 10.4 illustrates some physiological responses to cold exposure.

The effects of acclimation to the cold are less pronounced than those of acclimation to heat. However, athletes who train in the cold can become habituated to the cold, allowing their core temperature to drop slightly without causing shivering. People who are repeatedly exposed to the cold acclimate by increasing metabolic heat production, shivering more, and vasoconstricting more effectively. Behavioral adjustments are an important part of temperature regulation in the cold, as they are in the heat. Adding clothing, moving to a warmer spot, seeking shelter, and adjusting exercise intensity are common behavior adjustments.

Sweating during exercise in the cold can speed heat loss if the sweat soaks through clothing.

FIGURE 10.4 During exercise in the cold, the inside of an athlete's clothing can be a very warm place, so skin blood vessels dilate and sweating occurs. But when exercise stops or is reduced to a low intensity, core temperature can quickly fall below normal. When that occurs, the hypothalamus signals the sympathetic nervous system to constrict skin blood vessels (vasoconstrict) and also cause muscles to shiver. Those responses reduce heat loss and increase heat production.

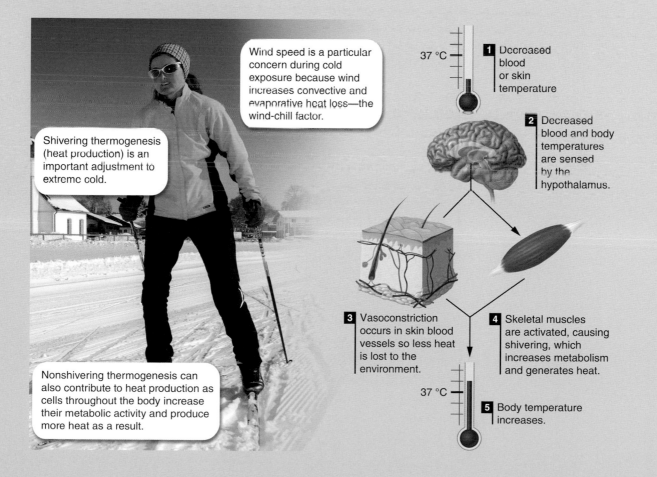

Wind speed is a particular concern during cold exposure because wind increases convective and evaporative heat loss—the wind-chill factor.

Shivering thermogenesis (heat production) is an important adjustment to extreme cold.

Nonshivering thermogenesis can also contribute to heat production as cells throughout the body increase their metabolic activity and produce more heat as a result.

1 Decreased blood or skin temperature

2 Decreased blood and body temperatures are sensed by the hypothalamus.

3 Vasoconstriction occurs in skin blood vessels so less heat is lost to the environment.

4 Skeletal muscles are activated, causing shivering, which increases metabolism and generates heat.

5 Body temperature increases.

Exposure to extreme or prolonged cold can overwhelm the body's attempts to maintain temperature. Whenever core temperature drops below normal, fewer motor units in muscle are recruited and the speed at which muscle cells shorten is reduced. Those two changes lessen power production, performance, and heat production. Shivering is an effective way for muscles to produce extra heat; but shivering requires ATP, which means that muscle glycogen stores can fall quickly. A normal response to exercise and to cold exposure is an increase in catecholamine hormone secretion. Epinephrine (adrenaline) and norepinephrine aid vasoconstriction and increase the release of free fatty acids from fat cells to help fuel shivering muscle cells. In very cold conditions, the vasoconstriction in fat cells actually reduces the release of fatty acids into the bloodstream, thereby reducing some of the fuel that muscle cells need for shivering.

Cold-water exposure is particularly dangerous to the body's ability to maintain temperature. In fact, heat loss in cold water is 4 times greater than in cold air, even when the body tries to slow heat loss by vasoconstricting skin blood vessels and increasing heat production through muscle contractions, increased metabolism, and shivering. As most people know from personal experience, being immersed in or sprayed with cold water can cause body temperature to drop quickly. Water has 26 times greater thermal conductivity than air, which means that being immersed in water accelerates heat loss from the body. Moving water increases heat loss further by convective cooling.

When core temperature drops below 94 °F (34.5 °C; *hypothermia*), the hypothalamus is not able to control temperature regulation and core temperature continues to drop. The colder the body becomes, the less able the hypothalamus is to control vasoconstriction and increase shivering. Heart rate slows, body temperature drops, drowsiness sets in, and with time coma and death become more likely.

Adapting to the cold involves cold habituation, metabolic acclimation, and insulative acclimation. It's no accident that cold-water swimmers carry extra body fat!

Exercise at Altitude

Chapter 3 mentions that the air you breathe is 21% oxygen (20.93%) and the rest is nitrogen, aside from a small amount of carbon dioxide. At sea level and low altitudes (lower than 1,500 ft, or 500 m), the atmospheric pressure is high enough to ensure that lungs are exposed to enough O_2 molecules so that breathing is easy, especially at rest. But on the highest place on Earth, Mt. Everest, the atmospheric pressure is only 33% of that at sea level. As a result, the O_2 molecules are spread so far apart that breathing becomes difficult because the oxygen content of blood is reduced. (Reduced atmospheric pressure is often referred to as *hypobaria* and reduced oxygen content in blood is called *hypoxia*.) Even though the air at the peak of Mt. Everest still contains 21% oxygen, the atmospheric pressure at 29,029 feet is very low because there is much less air above to create pressure. (See figure 10.5) At sea level, there is a 24-mile-high column of air pressing down on you. On Mt. Everest, that column of air is less than 19 miles high. At altitude, breathing has to be very rapid to introduce enough oxygen into the lungs to satisfy even the low metabolic needs at rest.

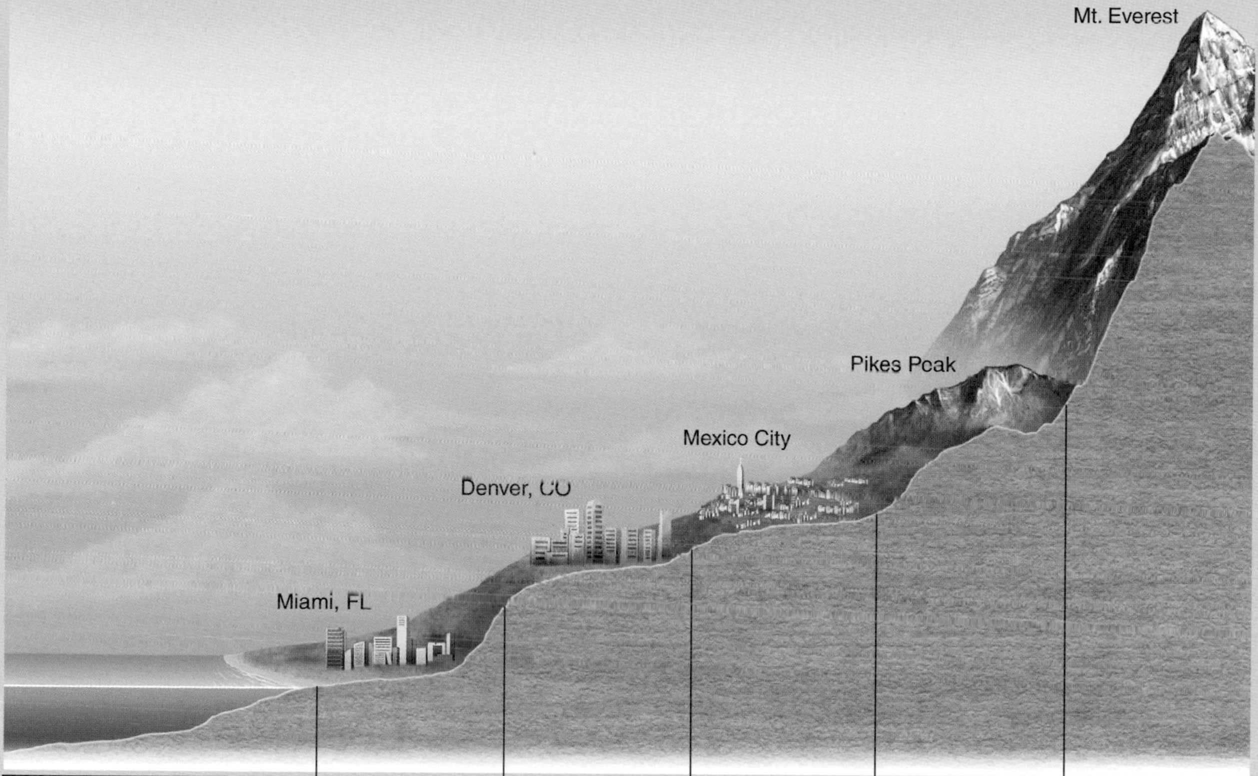

	0 (sea level)	5,202	7,251	14,108	29,028
Altitude (ft) (m)	0	1,610	2,210	4,300	8,048
Barometric pressure P_b (mmHg)	760	631	585	430	253
% O_2 in the air	20.93	20.93	20.93	20.93	20.93
Partial pressure of oxygen PO_2 (mmHg) in the air	159	132	122	90	53
Typical temperature (°C) (°F)	15 / 59	9 / 47	2 / 36	−11 / 12	−43 / −46

FIGURE 10.5 As altitude increases, the percentage of oxygen in the air remains the same but the barometric pressure falls, which reduces the partial pressure of oxygen to which lungs are exposed.

Reprinted, by permission, from W.L. Kenney, J.H. Wilmore, and D.L. Costill, 2015, *Physiology of sport and exercise*, 6th ed. (Champaign, IL: Human Kinetics), 271.

Exercise at altitude reduces performance capacity because maximal aerobic capacity and power are reduced as the result of lower partial pressure of oxygen. For purposes of describing the effects of altitude on the human body, elevations are categorized in this way:

Low altitude is 1,500 to 7,000 feet (500-2,000 m) above sea level.

Moderate altitude is 7,000 to 10,000 feet (2,000-3,000 m).

High altitude is 10,000 to 18,000 feet (3,000 to 5,500 m).

Extremely high altitude is more than 18,000 feet (>5,500 m).

Impaired performance can occur above 5,000 feet (1,500 m). In addition to the direct effects of lower atmospheric pressure, colder and drier air at elevation also take a toll. On average, air temperature drops by 1 °C with every 500 feet of elevation. And cold air is dry air, which increases respiratory fluid loss, contributing to dehydration. Figure 10.6 details the physiological adjustments that occur with acute altitude exposure.

At altitude for three weeks or more, a variety of physiological adaptations occur that improve ability to cope with the stress of altitude. (See figure 10.7.) The ability to train and compete at altitude improves after living at altitude, but those capacities remain reduced compared to living at sea level.

FIGURE 10.6 On first exposure to altitude, several physiological adjustments occur to help in coping with the reduced partial pressure of oxygen in the air.

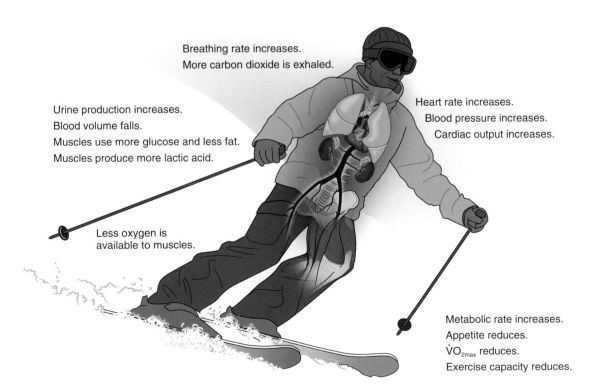

Breathing rate increases.
More carbon dioxide is exhaled.

Urine production increases.
Blood volume falls.
Muscles use more glucose and less fat.
Muscles produce more lactic acid.

Heart rate increases.
Blood pressure increases.
Cardiac output increases.

Less oxygen is available to muscles.

Metabolic rate increases.
Appetite reduces.
$\dot{V}O_{2max}$ reduces.
Exercise capacity reduces.

Does Training at Altitude Improve Performance at Sea Level?

At least three weeks of living at moderate altitude (7,000-10,000 ft, or 2133-3048 m) are needed for respiratory, cardiovascular, and muscle adaptations to occur. At higher altitudes, more time is needed. Those adaptations combine to improve the capacity for aerobic exercise at altitude. But do those adaptations help improve performance at sea level? The answer is no.

The likely reason that altitude training does not improve performance at sea level is that training intensity at altitude is reduced. In other words, a reduced training stimulus at altitude results in a reduced training response. Athletes are better-off training harder at lower altitudes and benefiting from the increased training stimulus. In addition, spending time at altitude leads to dehydration and loss of blood volume and muscle mass, all of which are bad for performance.

FIGURE 10.7 At altitude for three weeks or more, physiological adaptations occur that improve exercise capacity at altitude but not at sea level.

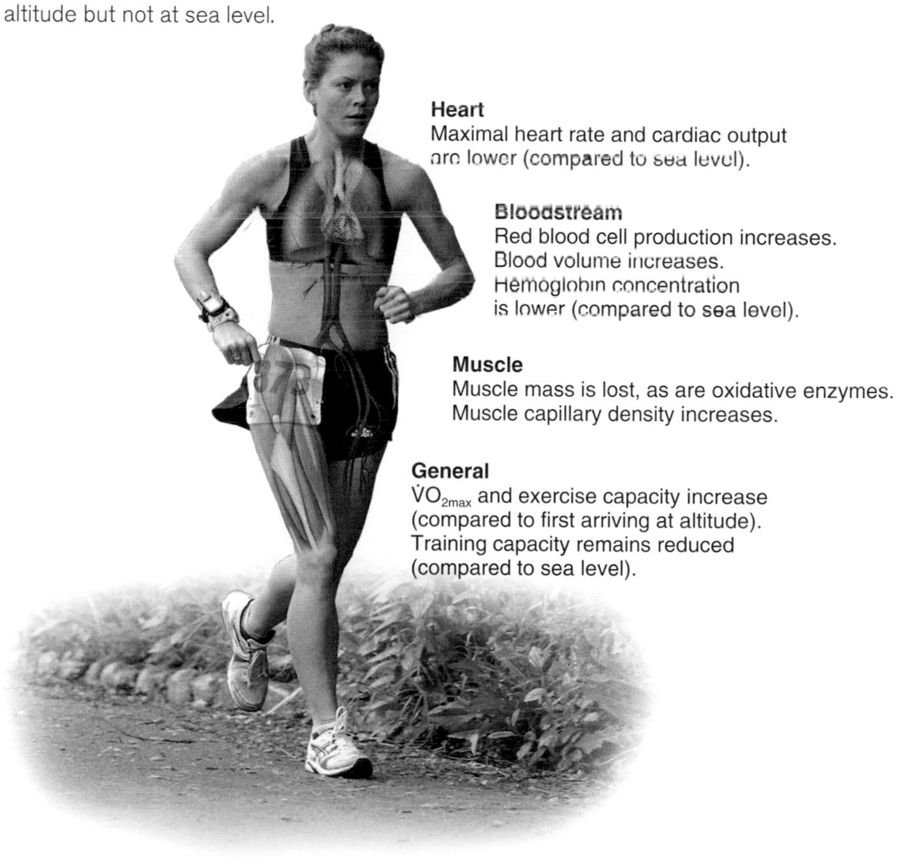

Heart
Maximal heart rate and cardiac output are lower (compared to sea level).

Bloodstream
Red blood cell production increases.
Blood volume increases.
Hemoglobin concentration is lower (compared to sea level).

Muscle
Muscle mass is lost, as are oxidative enzymes.
Muscle capillary density increases.

General
$\dot{V}O_{2max}$ and exercise capacity increase (compared to first arriving at altitude).
Training capacity remains reduced (compared to sea level).

Strategies for using altitude exposure as a way to improve performance both at altitude and closer to sea level depend on how much time the athlete can spend at altitude and whether the goal is to prepare for a competition at altitude or to use altitude-related adaptations to gain a competitive edge at sea level.

For a competition at altitude, arrive as soon as possible before the event so that there is not enough time for the adverse effects of altitude to occur. This option is best when competition is limited to one day. For competitions that are spread over a few days, the best strategy is to train at altitude for at least two weeks before the event so that adverse effects will have come and gone before competition. This approach is best suited for multiday events at altitude.

Perhaps the best approach for endurance athletes is to live at altitude to benefit from the adaptations but train at lower altitudes to maintain a high training stimulus and promote even greater adaptations. In short, live high, train low. Some athletes use hypoxic sleeping tents to simulate living at altitude to provoke increases in blood volume and hemoglo-

© Gorfer/iStock

bin that can benefit endurance performance. Research shows that living at 6,600 to 8,200 feet (2,000-2,500 m) seems to provoke the optimal responses.

Health Risks at Altitude

As many recreational skiers have experienced, taking a vacation at altitude can sometimes be a real headache. In fact, headaches are the most common symptom of altitude sickness, also known as acute mountain sickness. Six hours or more after arriving at altitude, headache, nausea, rapid breathing, and disturbed sleep can occur. After three or four days, the symptoms lessen or disappear. Higher altitudes provoke greater symptoms and in more people. In severe cases, physicians can prescribe medications to ease the symptoms.

While acute altitude sickness can knock vacationers off their skis for a few days, at higher altitudes the reactions can be life threatening, as shown in figure 10.8.

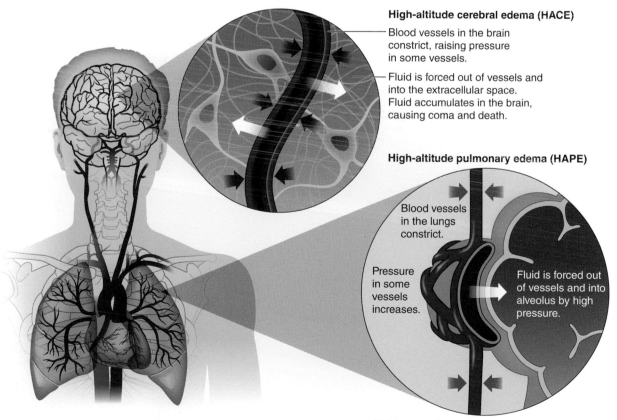

High-altitude cerebral edema (HACE)

Blood vessels in the brain constrict, raising pressure in some vessels.

Fluid is forced out of vessels and into the extracellular space. Fluid accumulates in the brain, causing coma and death.

High-altitude pulmonary edema (HAPE)

Blood vessels in the lungs constrict.

Pressure in some vessels increases.

Fluid is forced out of vessels and into alveolus by high pressure.

Fluid accumulates in lungs, causing difficulty in breathing and increased risk of clotting.

▌FIGURE 10.8   High-altitude sickness must be treated immediately.

CHAPTER ELEVEN

Training Children, Older Adults, and Pregnant Women

Maturation, age, and pregnancy influence the design of training programs.

Athletes and fitness clients come in all shapes, sizes, ages, and physical capacities, all with unique goals, interests, schedules, and challenges. Children, older adults, and pregnant women represent three categories of athletes and clients who present unique challenges for the design and implementation of effective training programs. Understanding how these individuals respond and adapt to physical activity and regular training is essential in designing programs that take into consideration the benefits and limitations associated with exercise.

Do Children Respond Differently Than Adults to Exercise Training?

Regular physical activity has lifelong benefits, regardless of a person's age. The human body is designed for movement, accomplishing physical tasks, and adapting to increased physical demands. You know that lack of physical activity at any time of life has negative implications for health, longevity, and quality of life. Sitting for hours at a desk or in front of a television or computer is associated with negative health outcomes that can be minimized simply by moving more often during each day. You also recognize that developing good physical activity habits early in life helps you sustain those habits as you age, especially during the challenging times of life when it often seems easier to forgo activity for other priorities. First and foremost, physical activity at any age should be fun because enjoyment is a strong motivator for continuing any behavior. For children, the joy of physical activity should be the centerpiece of their sport and fitness programs. But aside from the necessity of keeping things fun, it is important to recognize that, in many respects, children are not simply small adults. The ways in which children and adults differ in their responses to physical activity and training must be considered in designing training programs for children.

One example of the differences between adults and children is the large disparity often apparent between the ages of children and their maturity levels. Age and maturation are sometimes disconnected, especially when it comes to emotions and behavior. You know friends or children whom you consider to be more or less mature for their ages. But those judgments are made on the basis of whether or not their emotional reactions or behaviors fit expectations for a particular age.

From a physical perspective, maturation (maturity) is determined with a little more objectivity. People mature physically at slightly different rates from infancy (from birth to the first birthday), through childhood, and into adolescence, before finally reaching adulthood. (See figure 11.1.) At any given time in development, physical maturity is determined by

By age two, most children will have already reached 50% of their adult height.

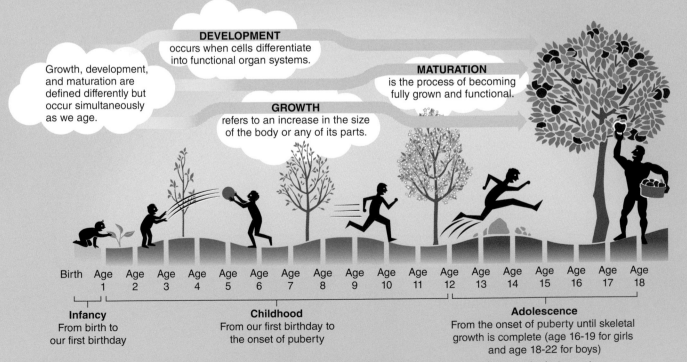

DEVELOPMENT occurs when cells differentiate into functional organ systems.

Growth, development, and maturation are defined differently but occur simultaneously as we age.

MATURATION is the process of becoming fully grown and functional.

GROWTH refers to an increase in the size of the body or any of its parts.

Birth | Age 1 | Age 2 | Age 3 | Age 4 | Age 5 | Age 6 | Age 7 | Age 8 | Age 9 | Age 10 | Age 11 | Age 12 | Age 13 | Age 14 | Age 15 | Age 16 | Age 17 | Age 18

Infancy
From birth to our first birthday

Childhood
From our first birthday to the onset of puberty

Adolescence
From the onset of puberty until skeletal growth is complete (age 16-19 for girls and age 18-22 for boys)

▌FIGURE 11.1 Growth, development, and maturation are defined differently but occur simultaneously during aging.

172

chronological age, skeletal age, and stage of sexual maturation.

In some sports, age-group competition is a common way to attempt to have children and adolescents compete against other kids of similar maturity. In other sports, body weight is used to categorize competitors to make competition more fair. Rules of this sort can help level the playing field but cannot account for different levels of maturity. For example, 10- to 12-year-old swimmers vary dramatically in height, weight, and sexual maturity. And there can be similarly large differences in the maturity of 14-year-old and 18-year-old wrestlers in the same weight class. Although only so much can be done to have competitions fairly reflect the differences that occur during aging, you have to keep those differences in mind when developing training programs.

Does Training Hurt or Help Children's Bones?

As with skeletal muscles and the heart, bone adapts to the stress imposed by regular exercise. Well-designed training programs, general play activities, and proper nutrition (adequate intake of calcium and vitamin D) stimulate adaptations that create stronger, healthier bones.

Most bones form from cartilage during fetal development, a process (*ossification*) that continues until the onset of adulthood. Bones grow as cartilage hardens into bone. The line of cartilage called the *epiphyseal plate* but commonly known as the *growth plate* indicates a bone that is still growing (figure 11.2). The growth plates in the bones of girls usually fuse a couple of years sooner than in boys' because female hormones signal the growth plates to close.

Regular physical activity at any age benefits bone health, but that is especially true in children and adolescents. High-impact activities such as running and repeated jumping stimulate bone formation by exposing the bone to sufficient stress to promote adaptations. *Bone mineral density* peaks during the 20s and then

gradually declines thereafter. Proper nutrition and exercise during adolescence create a greater peak bone density, an important factor in bone health throughout life. In women, menopause causes an accelerated loss of bone, increasing the risk of *osteoporosis* in those who had low bone density earlier in life.

Muscle mass typically peaks in girls between ages 16 and 20 and in boys between ages 18 and 25.

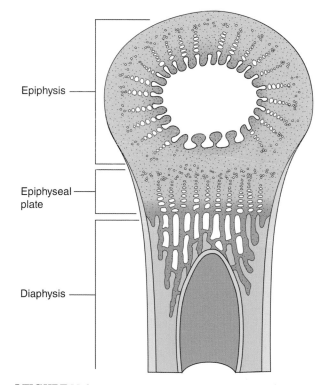

FIGURE 11.2 In children, the ends of long bones (such as the bones in the arms and legs) are made partly of cartilage. The bone grows as the cartilage hardens at the line called the growth plate or epiphyseal plate.

Epiphysis

Epiphyseal plate

Diaphysis

Development of the Nervous System

Regular physical activity—whether in organized sports or just playing in the yard—requires a child's developing nervous system to adapt to various demands. These adaptations occur year after year as the brain and motor nerves undergo *myelination.* (See figure 11.3.)

Regular physical activity helps children develop balance, agility, and coordination. For that reason, children should experience a variety of sports and activities so that they learn new skills and movement patterns and improve their fitness, responses that will benefit them throughout life. Motor skills improve rapidly through adolescence, another reason why it is important for children to participate in a variety of activities. Skills gained early in life are skills that can be used throughout life.

Blood pressure is related to body size and is lower in children than in adults.

FIGURE 11.3 The myelin sheath around nerve fibers develops during childhood and improves transmission of neural impulses.

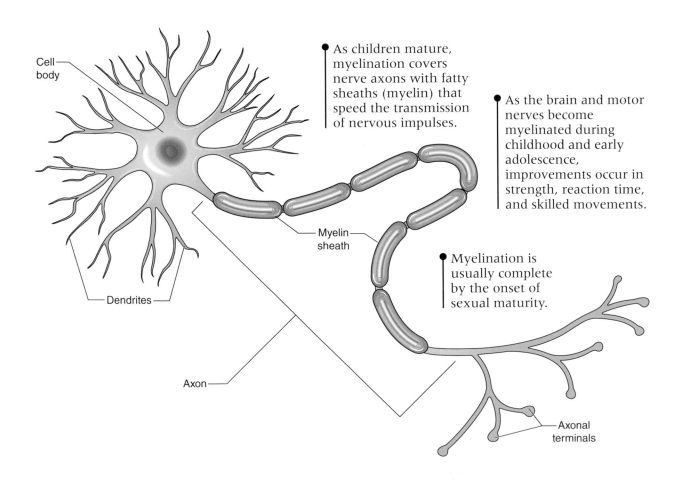

Cell body

As children mature, myelination covers nerve axons with fatty sheaths (myelin) that speed the transmission of nervous impulses.

As the brain and motor nerves become myelinated during childhood and early adolescence, improvements occur in strength, reaction time, and skilled movements.

Myelin sheath

Myelination is usually complete by the onset of sexual maturity.

Dendrites

Axon

Axonal terminals

Can Children Improve Strength With Training?

The short answer to this question is yes, children can increase their strength through proper training, including resistance exercise.

Strength increases during physical maturity because muscles naturally become larger. Not surprisingly, puberty sparks a rapid increase in muscle strength in both boys and girls. As growth slows toward the end of adolescence, muscle strength plateaus unless jobs or exercise routines stress muscles enough to stimulate the adaptations needed for increased strength.

Before puberty, increases in strength occur without any changes in the size of muscles. Keep in mind that strength can increase by the recruitment of more motor units, as a result of improved coordination, and through the development of better sport-specific skills, none of which require an increase in muscle size. All of the principles of training apply to children as they do to adults. However, extra care should be taken to prevent injury, especially with strength training. Following is an overview of recommendations.

Before puberty, strength gains are due to changes in the nervous system (better coordination, increased motor unit recruitment), with little to no change in muscle size.

Recommendations for Strength Training in Children

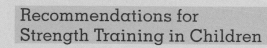

Proper exercise technique should always be the top priority, regardless of an athlete's age. This is particularly true with young athletes.

Progress from body-weight exercises to conventional strength training exercises using little to no weight to help kids learn proper technique.

Keep training volume low, keep the exercises simple, and gradually increase the number of exercises.

Eventually teach all the basic exercise and lifting techniques, which is something that should be accomplished over years, not months.

In teaching new techniques, always begin with little to no resistance.

As kids reach puberty, begin to transition from general resistance exercises to sport-specific resistance exercises.

After puberty, the volume and intensity of strength training can be gradually increased.

As an increasing number of children become overweight or obese, there is no doubt that increasing daily physical activity is an important part of stimulating weight loss. Current guidelines call for children to engage in at least 60 minutes of physical activity each day. The American Academy of Pediatrics recommends that overweight children increase their daily physical activity (energy output) and modestly restrict their energy intake by choosing a balanced diet of healthy foods, in appropriate portions, to produce a gradual loss of body weight (e.g., 1 lb/wk, or 0.5 kg/wk). It is always best to recommend that parents consult a pediatrician for guidance in helping their children lose fat weight.

How Do Children Respond to Exercise?

As children grow, so does the function of all physiological systems. Although children have immature physiological systems, they can participate in virtually all types of exercise without undue risk to health as long as the limitations in their physiology are taken into consideration. For example, children have a limited capacity for anaerobic exercise because their muscles contain low levels of anaerobic (glycolytic) enzymes. For that and other reasons, high-intensity training should wait until adolescence. Figure 11.4 illustrates how children respond to a single bout of exercise.

Should training programs be modified to account for how children adapt to training? The short answer is no. Although there are some differences between children and adults in the magnitude of the adaptations to training, children adapt to the stress of exercise training in similar ways. None of those differences are cause for altering the principles of training program design covered in chapter 5. Here are the expected responses to training in children:

- Children can decrease body weight and body fat, but their increase in lean body mass with training is less than in adolescents and adults.

- Muscle glycolytic capacity, PC, and ATP levels all increase with training in children.

- Regular training has no effect on the height achieved in adulthood.

- Improvements in $\dot{V}O_{2max}$ in children range from 5% to 15%, compared to 15% to 25% in adolescents and adults.

- The improvement in $\dot{V}O_{2max}$ after puberty may be due to increases in stroke volume that occur as the heart grows.

$\dot{V}O_{2max}$ and running economy are lower in children than in adults.

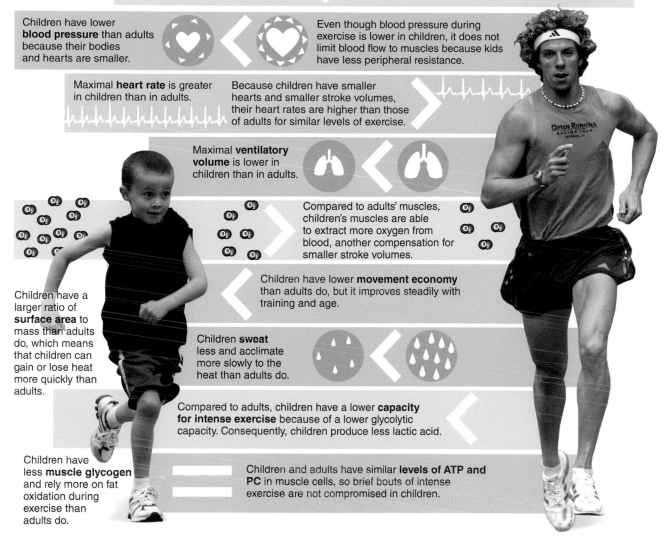

$\dot{V}O_{2max}$ is lower in children than in adults, but increases progressively with age until the end of adolescence.

$\dot{V}O_{2max}$ will increase with training but those changes are relatively small compared to the changes that adults undergo. However, performance improvements in children can be large.

Children have lower **blood pressure** than adults because their bodies and hearts are smaller.

Even though blood pressure during exercise is lower in children, it does not limit blood flow to muscles because kids have less peripheral resistance.

Maximal **heart rate** is greater in children than in adults.

Because children have smaller hearts and smaller stroke volumes, their heart rates are higher than those of adults for similar levels of exercise.

Maximal **ventilatory volume** is lower in children than in adults.

Compared to adults' muscles, children's muscles are able to extract more oxygen from blood, another compensation for smaller stroke volumes.

Children have lower **movement economy** than adults do, but it improves steadily with training and age.

Children have a larger ratio of **surface area** to mass than adults do, which means that children can gain or lose heat more quickly than adults.

Children **sweat** less and acclimate more slowly to the heat than adults do.

Compared to adults, children have a lower **capacity for intense exercise** because of a lower glycolytic capacity. Consequently, children produce less lactic acid.

Children have less **muscle glycogen** and rely more on fat oxidation during exercise than adults do.

Children and adults have similar **levels of ATP and PC** in muscle cells, so brief bouts of intense exercise are not compromised in children.

FIGURE 11.4 Although there are differences between children and adults in some of the physiological and metabolic responses to acute exercise, none of those differences prevents children from participating in virtually all types of exercise.

Are Dietary Supplements Safe for Children?

It is impossible to provide a blanket recommendation for supplement consumption by children because there are more than 50,000 supplements on the market, most of which do not have adequate evidence of safety or efficacy. Children and adults alike should be able to consume all of the essential nutrients by eating a balanced diet rich in fruits, vegetables, lean meats, grains, and dairy products. A low-dose multivitamin and mineral supplement can help ensure an adequate intake of micronutrients if parents are concerned that their children are not always eating as healthy a diet as they would like. Unless recommended by a physician, there is normally no reason that children should consume other dietary supplements, and that is particularly true for sport supplements such as creatine and beta-alanine.

What Are the Safe Limits for Training in Children?

Not much is known about how endurance training affects children because the topic has not been well studied. It is known that children can adapt to endurance training and can undergo significant improvements in endurance performance in sports such as swimming, running, and cycling. There are unresolved concerns about how endurance training in children might affect overall growth, bone development, onset of menses, risk of orthopedic injuries, socialization, and psychological development. In those regards, research has lagged behind practical experience because in many sports, swimming being a good example, young children often train for hours on a daily basis without any documented issues with growth and development. However, in designing training programs for children, you need to take care in ensuring that training and nutrition can best augment natural growth and development both physically and psychologically.

A general rule is that children can begin to train like adults in late adolescence, toward the end of musculoskeletal growth, when their bodies are better able to withstand the intensity, duration, and frequency of vigorous training. There is no doubt that some young gymnasts, swimmers, and runners undertake training programs that many adult athletes would find impossible to handle, seemingly without any long-term negative consequences. This is a good example of where the art and experience of training and coaching are often the best guides in making decisions about how hard, how long, and how often children should train, in part because there is not yet enough scientific information on which to base such decisions.

Can Older Adults Adapt to Training?

Now jump to the other end of the age spectrum and consider how older adults respond to exercise and adapt to training. The good news is that being physically active on a daily basis, along with periodic strength training, can slow or reverse many of the changes that occur during aging.

Changes With Aging

A variety of changes occur during the aging process, as shown in figure 11.5. For many, these changes can eventually interfere with daily activities such as opening jars, lifting groceries, and maintaining balance. Some of these changes are unavoidable, but most of them can be positively affected by regular physical activity and training.

Body weight tends to increase after age 25 because of reduction in physical activity and increase in energy (caloric) intake. After age 65, body weight tends to decrease as appetite and physical activity decline and muscle mass is lost. Loss of muscle mass can begin earlier if physical activity is reduced.

From a sport perspective, performance capacity is greatest during the 20s through early 30s and begins to decline slowly thereafter. The decline in distance and sprint performance averages about 1% each year after age 25. After age 60, the rate of decline increases to 2% per year. The reduction in performance capacity with aging is associated with the declines in strength and aerobic capacity. Although a decline in performance capacity is inevitable during aging, that decline can be slowed with regular training. In fact, sport performance in some older adults can equal or exceed that of many younger adults.

FIGURE 11.5 A variety of changes occur in the body during aging. In sedentary people, these changes are often more pronounced.

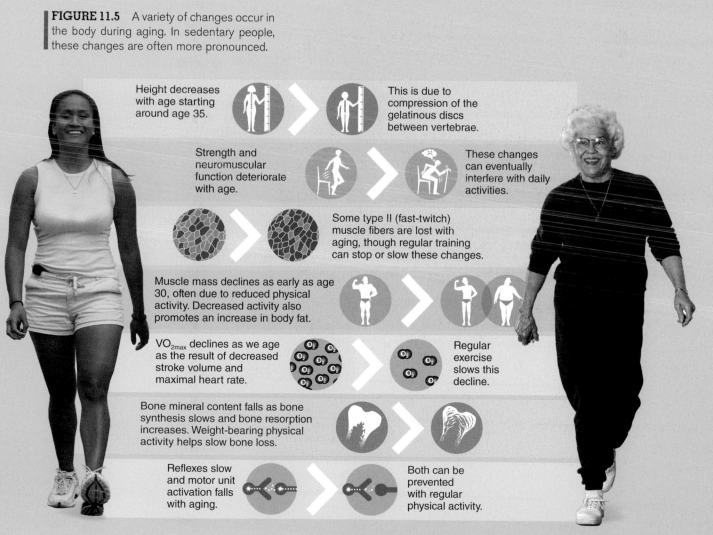

Height decreases with age starting around age 35.

This is due to compression of the gelatinous discs between vertebrae.

Strength and neuromuscular function deteriorate with age.

These changes can eventually interfere with daily activities.

Some type II (fast-twitch) muscle fibers are lost with aging, though regular training can stop or slow these changes.

Muscle mass declines as early as age 30, often due to reduced physical activity. Decreased activity also promotes an increase in body fat.

VO_{2max} declines as we age as the result of decreased stroke volume and maximal heart rate.

Regular exercise slows this decline.

Bone mineral content falls as bone synthesis slows and bone resorption increases. Weight-bearing physical activity helps slow bone loss.

Reflexes slow and motor unit activation falls with aging.

Both can be prevented with regular physical activity.

How Can Exercise Training Benefit Older Adults?

Older women and men respond to training similarly to younger people, increasing performance capacity along with physiological and metabolic function. For that reason, it is not unusual for 60-year-old athletes to have performance capacities that are greater than the capacities in people half their age. The ability to maintain impressive performance capacities occurs despite the fact that maximum cardiac output declines with age because both maximum heart rate and maximum stroke volume fall with age, as does blood flow to the arms and legs. It is difficult to separate the effects of aging from the effects of decades of relative inactivity and reduced training intensity and duration. However, the good news is that proper training clearly improves all facets of physical capacity, including muscle mass, strength, endurance, aerobic capacity, agility, balance, flexibility, and anaerobic capacity.

The loss of muscle mass and function associated with aging is called *sarcopenia*, a word coined in 1988 that means "poverty of flesh" in Greek. Regular strength training can help maintain muscle mass, strength, and neuromuscular function, even in very old adults. Figure 11.6 shows a strik-

> After age 60, the failure rate for opening the lid on a jar rises substantially.

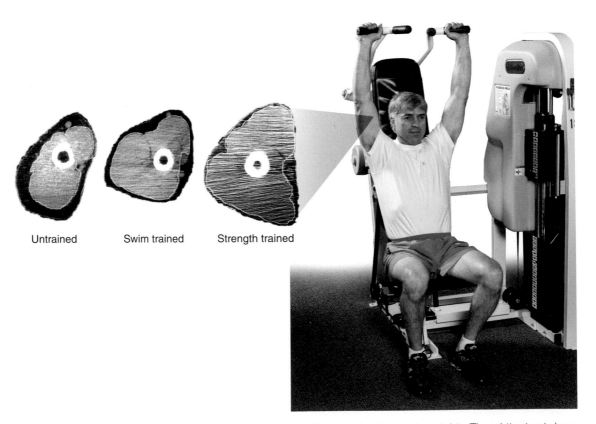

Untrained   Swim trained   Strength trained

FIGURE 11.6 Scans of the upper arms of three 57-year-old men of similar body weights. The white ring is bone, the gray area is muscle, and the black area is subcutaneous fat.

Reprinted, by permission, from W.L. Kenney, J.H. Wilmore, and D.L. Costill, 2015, *Physiology of sports and exercise*, 6th ed. (Champaign, IL: Human Kinetics), 453.

ing example of the effect of strength training on muscle mass in later middle age. Strength training can also slow the loss of type II muscle fibers, and physical activity that incorporates weight-bearing exercises such as running and jumping (impact exercise) helps slow bone loss. Reducing the loss of muscular strength and mass during aging is critical in maintaining the ability to live independently, decreasing the incidence of accidental falls, promoting more rapid recovery from injury and illness, and improving the overall quality of life.

Endurance training has no impact on the loss of muscle mass with age. Only strength training preserves muscle mass with age. However, endurance training helps slow the decline in $\dot{V}O_{2max}$ with age (figure 11.7).

Regular physical activity reduces the risk of early death and also lowers the risks associated with heat and cold exposure. Heat stress can be a particular problem for older adults, especially for those who are ill or have particularly low fitness. When older adults are exposed to heat stress, blood flow to the skin and sweating are less than in younger adults, causing core temperature to rise more quickly. Fortunately, aerobic training can improve blood flow to the skin, sweating, and the distribution of blood flow among skin, active muscles, and internal organs. With cold exposure, the blood vessels of the skin constrict less in older adults; because muscle mass is typically lower, older adults have a reduced ability to generate metabolic heat. These changes make older adults—especially the elderly—more susceptible to the cold. Adding more clothing when exercising outdoors and making other minor accommodations may be necessary for compensating for these age-related declines.

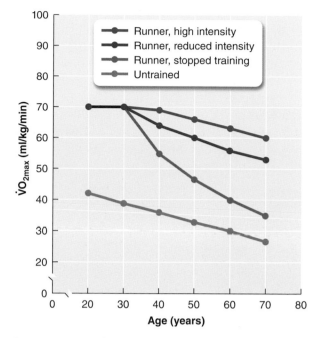

FIGURE 11.7 Runners who had a high level of aerobic fitness early in life and continue intense training as they age maintain a high level of fitness, even though they have some overall decline in fitness. Even if they reduce intensity or stop training, however, their fitness remains higher than that of people who had never trained.

Reprinted, by permission, from W.L. Kenney, J.H. Wilmore, and D.L. Costill, 2015, *Physiology of sport and exercise*, 6th ed. (Champaign, IL: Human Kinetics), 471.

Exercise is important during the aging process because it preserves and protects mitochondria. Exercise helps keep mitochondria young.

Training Program Tips for Older Adults

The U.S. Centers for Disease Control and Prevention (CDC) guidelines for physical activity also apply to older adults and can be used as a general framework in creating and tailoring training programs for older adults.

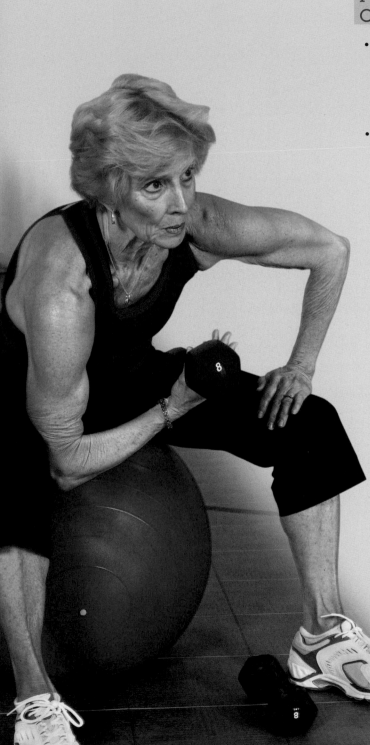

Physical Activity Guidelines for Older Adults

- Training programs for older adults should emphasize basic aerobic conditioning; exercises to improve muscular strength and mass; and activities that enhance flexibility, balance, and agility.

- Complete at least 2 hours 30 minutes of moderate physical activity (e.g., brisk walking) plus strength training at least twice each week to work all the major muscle groups.

- For those able to tackle more vigorous activity, at least 1 hour 15 minutes of activity similar to jogging or running plus strength training twice each week are recommended.

- Even greater health benefits are associated with doubling the total weekly duration of exercise.

- Exercising as little as 10 minutes at a time is associated with improved function and health.

- Walking, bicycling, swimming, and other activities of a continuous nature are good starting points for improving aerobic capacity.

- Simple body-weight exercises such as wall push-ups, toe stands, seated knee extensions, standing knee curls, supine pelvic tilts, and prone back extensions are examples of resistance exercises that can improve functional capacity and muscular strength. These exercises can help older adults prepare for more strenuous resistance training with exercise bands, free weights, and other equipment or simply as a way to continue exercising at home.

- Fitness classes of any sort, including yoga, are also appropriate for suitably motivated older adults.

Should Women Exercise During Pregnancy?

The American College of Sports Medicine (ACSM) encourages women to exercise throughout pregnancy as long as there are no contraindications. Regular exercise during normal pregnancies reduces health risks for both mother and baby, and the physiological changes that accompany training—such as increased blood volume—help support continued physical activity. Training programs for pregnant women should be modified to suit each woman's interests, abilities, and symptoms. Following are general guidelines for exercise for pregnant women, but women should always consult their physicians for individual advice on the proper exercise program.

Pregnant women need to consume an extra 300 Calories per day to support the developing fetus, so women who train during pregnancy should pay particular attention to adequate energy intake.

Training Guidelines for Pregnant Women

- Recommended exercise includes activities that use large muscle groups, such as walking, cycling, and swimming.
- During the first trimester, exercise can start at 15 minutes per day 3 days per week or as comfort and symptoms dictate.
- After the first trimester, exercise should be limited to 30 minutes per day 4 days per week at a moderate intensity (e.g., heart rate less than 155 bpm).
- Avoid dry-land supine exercise after the 16th week of pregnancy to reduce the risk of venous obstruction.
- Avoid hot environments and remain well hydrated.
- Strength training can be continued during pregnancy using resistance that results in modest fatigue after 12 to 15 reps.
- Never restrict breathing during exercise (i.e., no Valsalva maneuvers).
- Contraindications for exercise during pregnancy include anemia, diabetes, bronchitis, obesity, anorexia, hypertension, joint pain or injury, uncontrolled seizures, heart and lung disease, bleeding, and premature labor.
- Exercise can resume about a month after vaginal delivery and 2 months after cesarean section.

Menstruation, Hormones, and Exercise Performance

Although still a matter of some debate among sport scientists, menstruation does not seem to affect physiological and metabolic responses to exercise, nor does it influence sport performance, unless the symptoms are so severe as to restrict exercise. In fact, world records across sports have been set during every phase of the menstrual cycle. There is no doubt that menstruation and its hormonal underpinnings influence body temperature, fluid balance, and metabolism, but the combined effects of those changes on performance are less clear.

The age at which menstruation occurs (*menarche*) does not seem to be affected by the type of sport. Small, lean girls in any sport are most likely to have delayed menarche because of low body fat. Disturbances in the menstrual cycle (e.g., infrequent or no periods) in athletes and nonathletes alike can occur with caloric restriction. This energy deficit can be exaggerated in athletes because of the large daily energy outputs associated with training. Energy deficits in female athletes can affect long-term health of bones and reproductive organs because of reductions in estrogen, progesterone, luteinizing hormone, and thyroid production along with compromised intakes of calcium, vitamin D, and protein.

One of the reasons that girls are at increased risk of injury to the anterior cruciate ligament (ACL) compared to boys is that testosterone strengthens ligaments, whereas estrogen (and perhaps other hormones) weakens ligaments. When the fibroblasts in ligaments are exposed to testosterone, they increase their production of collagen proteins, strengthening the ligaments. Estrogen exposure decreases collagen production. Other factors that increase the risk of ACL injuries in girls include differences in quadriceps and hamstring strength as well as differences in the biomechanics of how girls land after jumping. For these reasons, training in young girls should stress leg-strength exercises and proper landing techniques, especially in sports such as basketball, soccer, softball, lacrosse, and hockey.

INDEX OF COMMON QUESTIONS FROM CLIENTS

General Physiology

What makes a muscle contract? (chapter 1, p. 6)

How do nerves talk to muscles? (chapter 1, p. 6)

Why do muscles feel tight when I stretch? (chapter 1, 11)

Are there different types of muscle fibers? Do some people have more of one type than the other? (chapter 1, p. 10)

What causes fatigue? (chapter 4, p. 62)

Why am I sore the day after a workout? (chapter 1, p. 18)

Does lactic acid cause fatigue? (chapter 4, p. 69)

What's the difference between aerobic and anaerobic metabolism? (chapter 2, p. 29)

How does oxygen get into the bloodstream? (chapter 3, p. 46)

Will exercise change my blood pressure? (chapter 3, p. 56)

What separates great athletes from the rest of us? (chapter 8, p. 129)

Is a loss of physical ability with aging inevitable? (chapter 11, p. 179)

What causes muscles to cramp? (chapter 1, p 19)

Program Design

Why does the same training program have different effects on different people? (chapter 1, p. 13; chapter 5, p. 81; chapter 9, p. 143)

What makes a good training program? (chapter 5, p. 80)

If I stop training, will I lose all of my gains in fitness? (chapter 5, p. 83)

What is overtraining? (chapter 4, p. 72; chapter 5, p. 84)

How can I tell if I'm overtraining? (chapter 4, p. 73; chapter 5, p. 90)

Should I cross-train? (chapter 8, p. 135)

When it comes to exercise, how are children different from adults? (chapter 11, p. 172)

Should older adults exercise the same way that younger adults would? (chapter 11, p. 182)

Should women exercise during pregnancy? (chapter 11, p. 183)

Strength Training and Hypertrophy

What changes in my body when I do strength training? (chapter 1, p. 17)

Why do muscles get stronger when I train? (chapter 1, p. 20)

What makes muscles get bigger? (chapter 1, p. 20)

What determines how much muscle I can gain? (chapter 6, p. 94)

Will lifting weights give women big, bulky muscles? (chapter 6, p. 96)

How often should I strength-train, and how many sets should I do?
  (chapter 6, p. 98)

Can I build strength if I have only a short time for a workout?
  (chapter 6, p. 100)

What kinds of equipment are best for strength training? (chapter 6, p. 98)

Does muscle damage lead to increased strength? (chapter 1, p. 18)

What are the effects of steroids on the body? (chapter 6, p. 101)

Should endurance athletes strength-train? (chapter 9, p. 151)

Endurance Training

What changes in my body when I do aerobic training?
  (chapter 1, p. 14; chapter 3, p. 48; chapter 9, p. 140)

Will aerobic fitness help my long-term health? (chapter 9, p. 141)

Why do target heart rate and maximum heart rate get lower with age?
  (chapter 3, p. 52)

What is $\dot{V}O_{2max}$? (chapter 3, p. 50)

What is the relationship between $\dot{V}O_{2max}$ and endurance performance?
  (chapter 9, p. 142)

What is the lactate threshold? (chapter 9, p. 145)

How should I plan my training for an endurance event? (chapter 9, p. 148)

How long will my endurance keep improving with training?
  (chapter 3, p. 51)

Does endurance training give you more red blood cells? (chapter 9, p. 147)

Is endurance important for athletes in team sports and nonendurance
  events? (chapter 9, p. 152)

Why do East African runners win so many endurance events?
  (chapter 9, p. 144)

Anaerobic and Interval Training

What changes in my body when I do anaerobic training? (chapter 1, p. 16)

What is interval training? (chapter 8, p. 130)

How can I incorporate interval training into my workout?
  (chapter 8, p. 130)

Should I do high-intensity interval training (HIIT)? How often?
  (chapter 5, p. 81)

Can high-intensity interval training increase my endurance?
(chapter 9, p. 148)

What are the benefits of plyometric training? (chapter 8, p. 134)

What does *power* really mean in athletic events? (chapter 8, p. 126)

Weight Loss and Metabolism

Why do I have a difficult time losing weight? (chapter 7, p. 118)

How many Calories do I need to eat each day? (chapter 7, p. 114)

What factors affect how many Calories I burn in a day? (chapter 7, p. 109)

How many Calories do common physical activities burn? (chapter 7, p. 112)

Does consuming Calories during my workout defeat the purpose of trying to lose weight? (chapter 7, p. 123)

How can I lose fat without losing muscle? (chapter 7, p. 120)

What's the best way to lose abdominal fat? (chapter 7, p. 121)

What is the best exercise intensity for burning fat? (chapter 7, p. 122)

Will I burn more fat if I work out while fasting or on a low-carbohydrate diet? (chapter 7, p. 124)

What does it mean to have a fast metabolism? How can I speed up my metabolism? (chapter 3, p. 50)

What is my resting metabolic rate? (chapter 7, p. 114)

What is the oxygen deficit? Am I still burning extra Calories after my workout? (chapter 3, p. 53)

What is brown fat? (chapter 7, p. 110)

Should children diet? (chapter 11, p. 176)

Safety and Environmental Issues

How can I avoid muscle cramps? (chapter 1, p. 19)

Why is it so much harder to exercise when it is hot? (chapter 10, p. 156)

What are the risks of exercising in the heat? (chapter 10, p. 160)

What precautions should I take when exercising in the heat? (chapter 10, p. 157)

Will acclimating to the heat improve my performance? (chapter 10, p. 158)

Why is hydration important?
(chapter 2, p. 42; chapter 4, p. 67; chapter 10, p. 156)

Is it possible to drink too much? (chapter 2, p. 44)

Should I drink during cold-weather activity? (chapter 10, p. 166)

Why do I feel weaker when I'm at altitude? (chapter 10, p. 165)

Is there less oxygen at higher altitudes? (chapter 10, p. 165)

At what altitude is exercise performance affected? (chapter 10, p. 166)

Does training at altitude improve performance at sea level?
(chapter 10, p. 167)

What exercises are safe for pregnant women? (chapter 11, p. 183)

Does menstruation affect exercise performance? (chapter 11, p. 184)

Is exercise training dangerous for children's growth? (chapter 11, p. 176)

Is it safe for children to strength-train? (chapter 11, p. 175)

Nutrition, Hydration, and Supplements

What do carbohydrate, fat, and protein do in my body? (chapter 2, p. 27)

What happens to carbohydrate after I eat it? (chapter 2, p. 32)

What happens to fat after I eat it? (chapter 2, p. 33)

What happens to protein after I eat it? (chapter 2, p. 35)

How much protein do I need to eat each day?
  (chapter 2, p. 34; chapter 6, p. 105)

Should I ingest protein after a workout?
  (chapter 2, p. 35; chapter 6, p. 105)

If I consume carbohydrate during my workout, will I avoid fatigue?
  (chapter 4, p. 66)

Will energy drinks improve my performance? (chapter 2, p. 37)

How much water do I need to drink each day? (chapter 2, p. 41)

What are the effects of dehydration? (chapter 4, p. 66)

Should I take high doses of vitamins and minerals? (chapter 2, p. 40)

What does iron do in the body, and what are the effects of not getting
  enough iron? (chapter 3, p. 47)

What dietary supplements can improve my speed and power?
  (chapter 8, p. 137)

What supplements can help me lose weight? (chapter 7, p. 114)

If muscles use ATP for energy, should I take an ATP supplement?
  (chapter 2, p. 24)

Note: The italicized *f* and *t* following page numbers refer to figures and tables, respectively.

A

abdominal fat 121
acclimation
    altitude 166-168, 166*f*, 167*f*
    cold 163, 164
    heat 158, 158*f*
acetaminophen 102
acetylcholine (ACh) 7*f*, 8
acidosis, metabolic 62*t*, 69-70, 69*f*.
    See also anaerobic training;
    lactic acid
actin 4*f*, 5, 7*f*, 8*f*, 9, 11, 12, 20, 22*f*,
    70*f*, 94, 95, 102
activity energy expenditure 49, 109*f*,
    112-113, 112*t*, 113*f*
acute mountain sickness 169, 169*f*
adaptation 87, 91, 129
adenosine triphosphate (ATP)
    depletion and fatigue 62, 62*t*, 63,
        63*f*
    energy systems and production
        28-30, 28*f*, 38, 38*f*, 38*t*, 53*f*
    makeup and breakdown 24-25,
        24*f*
    nutrient sources 26, 27, 27*f*, 29,
        30-33, 31*f*, 32*f*, 33*f*, 34, 36-37,
        36*f*, 37*f*, 40
    plant photosynthesis 23, 45, 108
    uses 24, 25
adolescence 172, 172*f*, 173, 174,
    174*f*, 175, 176, 177*f*, 178
adrenaline 52, 53, 89, 164
aerobic endurance. *See also* altitude
    defining 91
    gender differences 143
    muscle fiber characteristics of
        endurance athletes 10-11,
        10*f*, 11*t*
    nutrition and hydration consid-
        erations 34, 35, 37, 44, 65
    performance enhancement tech-
        niques 58-59, 147
    performance factors 13, 144,
        146, 146*f*
    training
        adaptations 12-13, 12*f*, 14-15,
            20, 54
        average energy cost across
            activities and equipment 49,
            112-113, 112*t*
        children 178
        Fartlek training 131, 149, 150
        guidelines 82, 148-150
        health benefits 140-141, 141*f*
        interval training 16, 81, 82,
            130, 131-133, 149, 150, 176
        lactate threshold 51, 57, 145,
            145*f*, 180
        older adults 181, 181*f*, 182
        sprinters and team-sport ath-
            letes 126, 152

strength training consider-
    ations 135, 148, 149, 151
tapering 89, 92, 149
V̇O$_{2max}$
    children 176, 177*f*
    gender differences 57, 143
    genetics 13, 57, 143
    lactate threshold connection
        51, 57, 145, 145*f*, 180
    limiting factors 13, 56, 57,
        140, 143
    measures and meaning 49,
        50, 139, 140-141
    older adults 179, 179*f*, 180,
        181, 181*f*
    performance enhancement
        techniques 58-59
    testing 51
    training 49, 50, 50*f*, 51, 54,
        55*f*, 56-57, 142, 142*f*
V̇O$_{2peak}$ 53
aerobic production of ATP 28, 28*f*,
    29, 38, 38*f*, 38*t*, 47, 53*f*
African distance runners 144
agility 91, 174, 180, 182
aging
    children 172-173, 172*f*
    older adults 50, 52, 105-106,
        179-182, 179*f*, 180*f*, 181*f*
altitude
    acclimation 59, 166-168, 166*f*,
        167*f*
    African runners 144
    breathing and oxygen supply 45,
        59, 165, 165*f*
    elevation and effects on perfor-
        mance 166, 166*f*
    health risks 169, 169*f*
    performance enhancement tents
        59, 168
American Academy of Pediatrics 176
American College of Sports Medicine
    (ACSM) 183
amino acids. *See* protein
amphetamines 71, 114
anabolic resistance 105
anabolic steroids 22, 22*f*, 101, 101*f*
anaerobic glycolysis 28, 28*f*, 29, 38,
    38*f*, 38*t*, 53*f*
anaerobic threshold 51, 57, 145,
    145*f*, 180. *See also* lactic acid
anaerobic training
    adaptations 16
    children 176, 177*f*
    endurance capacity connection
        152
    glycogen depletion 64, 65
    high-intensity interval training
        (HIIT) 16, 81, 82, 131, 132,
        149, 150, 176

monitoring intensity 133
anemia 47, 183
anterior cruciate ligament (ACL)
    injuries 134*f*, 184
anti-inflammatory drugs 102
axons 6*f*, 7*f*, 174*f*

B

balance 102, 174, 179, 180, 182
barometric pressure 45, 59, 165, 165*f*
basal metabolic rate (BMR) 49, 50
basketball 112, 112*t*, 135, 184. *See*
    also speed and power training
beta-alanine 137, 177
Bikram yoga 162
block periodization 84. *See also* peri-
    odization
blood and blood vessel function
    blood flow restriction and
        strength training 59, 104
    oxygen and carbon dioxide trans-
        port 46-47, 46*f*, 47*f*, 56
    red blood cells 46*f*, 47*f*, 57, 58,
        59 147
    training adaptations 54, 57, 88
blood doping 58, 147
blood pressure 15, 55*f*, 56, 59, 101,
    141*f*, 174, 177*f*, 183
body weight. *See* weight management
bone health
    adaptations to training 16, 17
    children 173, 173*f*, 178
    older adults 179*f*
    plyometric training 134*f*, 173
brain
    cardiovascular system function
        55*f*
    development in children 174,
        174*f*
    glucose 30, 66
    transmission disruption and
        fatigue 62, 62*t*, 71, 71*f*
breakfast 65, 120
breathing. *See* oxygen; Valsalva
    maneuvers
B vitamins 40, 40*t*

C

caffeine 37, 114
calcium 7*f*, 8, 8*f*, 9, 40, 70
Calories. *See also* nutrition; weight
    management
    energy balance versus energy
        availability 108-109, 108*f*,
        116-117, 117*t*, 179
    energy efficiency versus energy
        deficiency 109*f*, 110-111,
        116, 117*t*, 184
    estimating daily energy needs 50,
        114, 115, 115*t*
    fats and carbohydrates 53
    input 108, 108*f*, 109, 183

Calories *(continued)*
output 49, 50, 109-114, 109*f*, 110*f*, 112*t*, 113*f*, 115, 115*t*, 119, 120
severe restriction 114, 116, 119, 120
storage 37, 37*f*
capsaicin 19
carbohydrate
breakdown and uses in the body 26, 27, 27*f*, 29, 30-32, 31*f*, 32*f*, 36*f*, 38, 38*f*, 38*t*, 47
diet 64-65
hypoglycemia 62*f*, 65, 66
ingesting during exercise 123, 123*f*
recovery guidelines 99
respiratory exchange ratio (RER) 52-53
synthesis 23, 108
carbon dioxide
air composition 45
ATP production 29, 46
exchange for oxygen 46, 46*f*, 47, 47*f*, 48*f*
cardiac output. *See also* heart function
adaptations to training 14, 48, 54, 140
aerobic endurance capacity 56, 140, 142*f*
affecting factors 62*t*, 66, 89, 159*f*, 166*f*, 167*f*
aging 52, 180
dehydration 43, 129, 133, 161
cartilage 173, 173*f*
children
dieting and supplements 176, 177
maturation, growth, and development 172-175, 172*f*, 173*f*, 174*f*
training 172, 175, 176, 177f, 178
chocolate milk 35, 99
circuit training 131
citric acid cycle 28, 28*f*, 29, 38, 38*f*, 38*t*, 47, 53*f*
coffee 37, 114
colas 37, 114
cold
altitude 166
older adults 181
performance and acclimation effects 163-164, 163*f*
compression clothing 104
concentric contractions and training 9, 18, 102, 103*f*
conduction 156, 156*f*, 164. *See also* heat
convection 156, 156*f*, 164. *See also* heat
cooling aids 69, 157, 161, 162
coordination
developing 82, 174, 175
fatigue and overtraining 62*t*, 72*f*, 74, 152
core strength 133
cramps 19, 160-161
creatine 63, 106, 137, 177

cross-training 17, 135
cyclists 11*t*, 58, 89, 112*t*, 178
D
dairy 35, 99
dehydration. *See also* heat
altitude exposure 166, 167
effects 12, 19, 42-43, 62*t*, 66-67, 67*f*, 129, 133, 147, 156
fluid-regulatory mechanisms 41-42, 43, 158*f*
guidelines for fluid intake 40, 43, 44, 67
hyperthermia 66, 68, 68*f*, 156, 158*f*, 160-161, 162
hyponatremia 44
delayed-onset muscle soreness (DOMS) 18, 18*f*, 21, 21*f*, 102
dendrites 6*f*, 7*f*
Denver (Colorado) 165*f*
designing training programs. *See* program design
detraining 21, 21*f*, 80, 83, 83*f*
development 172-173, 172*f*
diastolic pressure 56. *See also* blood pressure
diet. *See* nutrition; weight management
diffusion coefficient 46
disease and illness 21, 21*f*, 129
disordered eating 114, 116, 119
distance runners 10, 10*f*, 11*t*, 28, 28*f*, 126, 144. *See also* running
DNA. *See* genetics
doping
blood doping 58, 147
steroids 22, 22*f*, 101, 101*f*
duration 91
E
eating disorders 114, 116, 119
eccentric muscle activity
delayed-onset muscle soreness (DOMS) 18, 18*f*, 21, 21*f*, 102
eccentric training 18, 82, 102, 103*f*, 134, 134*f*
titin 9, 11
economy of movement 143, 144, 146, 146*f*, 176, 177*f*
edema 18
elderly 179-182, 179*f*, 180*f*, 181*f*
electrical stimulation 104
electrolytes 19, 40. *See also* sport drinks
electron transport chain 28, 28*f*, 29, 38, 38*f*, 38*t*, 47, 54
endomysium 4*f*, 5
endurance. *See also* altitude
defining 91
muscle fiber characteristics of endurance athletes 10-11, 10*f*, 11*t*
nutrition and hydration considerations 34, 35, 37, 44, 65
performance enhancement techniques 58-59, 147
performance factors 13, 144, 146, 146*f*
training

adaptations 12-13, 12*f*, 14-15, 20, 54
average energy cost across activities and equipment 49, 112-113, 112*t*
children 178
Fartlek training 131, 149, 150
guidelines 82, 148-150
health benefits 140-141, 141*f*
high-intensity interval training (HIIT) 16, 81, 82, 131, 132, 149, 150, 176
interval training 130, 131-133
lactate threshold 51, 57, 145, 145*f*, 180
older adults 181, 181*f*, 182
power and speed training considerations 126
sprinters and team-sport athletes 152
strength training considerations 135, 148, 149, 151
tapering 89, 92, 149
$\dot{V}O_{2max}$
children 176, 177*f*
lactate threshold connection 51, 57, 145, 145*f*, 180
limiting factors 13, 56, 57, 140, 143
measures and meaning 49, 50, 139, 140-141
older adults 179, 179*f*, 180, 181, 181*f*
performance enhancement techniques 58-59
testing 51
training adaptations 50, 50*f*, 51, 54, 55*f*, 142, 142*f*
$\dot{V}O_{2peak}$ 53
energy. *See* adenosine triphosphate (ATP); Calories
energy drinks and bars 30, 32, 37, 65, 123
energy systems 28-30, 28*f*, 38, 38*f*, 38*t*, 53*f*. *See also* nutrition
environment. *See* altitude; cold; heat
enzymes
adaptations to training 12, 14, 16, 20, 54, 87, 132
ATP production 9, 24*f*, 25, 38
food to energy 30-31, 32, 34
function and production of enzymes 5, 35*f*, 39, 40
limiting factors on performance 47, 102, 167*f*
steroids and NSAIDs 101, 102
$\dot{V}O_{2max}$ 56, 142*f*
epimysium 4*f*, 5
epinephrine 52, 53, 89, 164
epiphyseal plate 173, 173*f*
erythropoietin (EPO) 58, 59, 147
estrogen 96, 184
excess postexercise oxygen consumption (EPOC) 53, 53*f*, 109*f*
exercise physiology 3

F

Fartlek training 131, 149, 150
fast-twitch muscle fibers
    adaptations to training 16
    characteristics and function
      10-11, 10*f*, 11*t*
    older adults 179*f*, 181
fat. *See also* weight management
    abdominal fat 121
    breakdown and uses in the body
      26, 27, 27*f*, 30, 32, 33*f*, 36*f*, 38,
      38*f*, 38*t*, 47
    respiratory exchange ratio (RER)
      52-53
    synthesis 23, 108
fat-free mass (FFM) 117, 117*t*
fatigue
    defining 61, 72, 91, 98
    glycogen depletion 62*t*, 64-65,
      64*f*, 65*f*
    hyperthermia 62*t*, 68, 68*f*, 69,
      160-161
    hypoglycemia 62*t*, 65, 66
    hypovolemia 12, 19, 42-43, 62*t*,
      66-67, 67*f*, 133, 147, 156, 166,
      167
    metabolic acidosis 62*t*, 69-70, 69*f*
    nervous system disruption 62,
      62*t*, 71, 71*f*
    overtraining 72-74, 72*f*, 73*f*, 75,
      84, 85, 85*f*, 89-90, 91
    PCR and ATP depletion 62, 62*t*,
      63, 63*f*
    training adaptations and effects
      on performance 75, 152
female athletes and exercisers
    anemia and energy deficits 47,
      184
    calcium needs and bone health
      40, 173
    hydration and hematocrit 41, 57,
      147
    increasing strength without mass
      13, 96, 96*f*
    jumping and knee injuries 134*f*,
      184
    perceptions of weight and fat
      storage 121
    pregnancy and training 183
    $\dot{V}O_{2max}$ differences across genders
      57, 143
fiber 31. *See also* carbohydrate
Fick equation 54
first law of thermodynamics 108
flexibility 11, 13, 135, 146*f*, 148, 162,
    180, 182
fluid intake. *See* hydration
fluoxetine 114
food. *See* nutrition
force 126, 128
forskolin 114
free weights 102, 103*f*
fructose 30, 31*f*, 32*f*
fuel. *See* adenosine triphosphate
    (ATP); Calories

G

galactose 30, 31*f*, 32*f*
garcinia cambogia 114

gels 30, 32, 123
gender differences
    anemia and energy deficits in
      females 47, 184
    calcium and bone growth 40, 173
    hydration and hematocrit 41, 57,
      147
    jumping and knee injuries 134*f*,
      184
    muscular training adaptations
      13, 96, 96*f*
    perceptions of weight and fat
      storage 121
    pregnancy and training 183
    $\dot{V}O_{2max}$ 57, 143
genetics
    ethnicity and endurance perfor-
      mance 144
    muscles 11, 12*f*, 94, 94*f*
    training response speed and mag-
      nitude 12-13, 12*f*, 81, 81*f*, 99,
      128, 129, 143
    $\dot{V}O_{2max}$ 13, 57, 143
    weight management 118*f*, 119
glucose 30-32, 31*f*, 32*f*, 37, 37*f*, 65
glycogen
    depletion and fatigue 62*t*, 64-65,
      64*f*, 65*f*
    energy source 5, 26, 29, 37, 37*f*,
      177*f*
glycolysis 28, 28*f*, 29, 38, 38*f*, 38*t*, 53*f*
green tea extract 114
growth 172-173, 172*f*, 173*f*
growth hormone (GH) 22, 101
gymnastics 17, 178

H

Harris-Benedict equation 115*t*
health
    benefits of exercise 56, 140-141,
      141*f*, 181
    competitive success 129
    disease and illness 21, 21*f*, 129
    eating disorders 114, 116, 119
    risks at altitude 169, 169*f*
heart function. *See also* cardiac output
    aerobic training 14, 15, 48, 48*f*,
      54, 55*f*
    heart rate and overtraining 73,
      73*f*, 74, 90
    heart rate monitoring and inten-
      sity 133
    maximal heart rate 52, 133, 167*f*,
      177*f*, 180
    older adults 52, 180
heat. *See also* dehydration
    acclimation 158, 158*f*
    children 177*f*
    effects on performance 155, 156-
      157, 158
    heat illnesses 62*t*, 66, 68, 68*f*, 71,
      156, 160-162
    hot yoga 162
    older adults 181
    precooling aids 69, 157
    pregnancy 183
    production and loss 156, 157*f*,
      159-160, 159*f*
heat cramps 19, 160-161

heat exhaustion 160, 161
heatstroke 68, 71, 160, 161, 162
height 172, 176, 179*f*
helium 45
hematocrit 57, 147
hemoglobin 46*f*, 47, 53, 58, 59, 140,
    142*f*, 144, 167*f*, 168
heredity. *See* genetics
high-altitude cerebral edema (HACE)
    169*f*
high-altitude pulmonary edema
    (HAPE) 169*f*
high-intensity interval training
    (HIIT) 16, 81, 82, 131, 132,
    137, 149, 150, 176
high responders 13, 57, 81, 81*f*, 129,
    143. *See also* genetics
homeostatic compensation 119
hormones
    aging effects 52
    anabolic hormones 22, 22*f*, 96,
      101, 173
    cold exposure 164
    exercise response 53, 97, 106,
      111, 164
    female hormones 96, 134*f*, 184
    hunger and satiety hormones
      109, 118, 119
    illegitimate uses 22
    production and functioning 35*f*,
      39*f*
hot yoga 162
humidity 68, 68*f*, 156, 157, 160,
    161, 162
hydration. *See also* heat
    altitude exposure 166, 167
    cellular adaptation and function-
      ing 12, 99, 129
    dehydration effects 12, 19,
      42-43, 62*t*, 66-67, 67*f*, 129,
      133, 147, 156
    fluid-regulatory mechanisms
      41-42, 43, 158*f*
    guidelines for fluid intake 40, 43,
      44, 67
    hyponatremia 44
    sports drinks 30, 32, 37
    temperature regulation 156, 157,
      158*f*, 159*f*
    water 41, 41*f*, 44, 45
hydrogen 45, 69, 70, 70*f*. *See also*
    water
hypertension 15, 56, 59, 101, 141*f*,
    183. *See also* blood pressure
hyperthermia 62*t*, 66, 68, 68*f*, 69,
    71, 156, 157, 160-162. *See also*
    dehydration
hypertrophy. *See also* training prin-
    ciples
    delayed-onset muscle soreness
      (DOMS) 18, 18*f*, 21, 21*f*, 102
    equipment, exercises, and con-
      tractions 102, 103*f*
    factors that influence muscle
      mass 94, 94*f*
    gender considerations 13, 96, 96*f*
    general guidelines for resistance
      training 98-99

hypertrophy *(continued)*
>   gimmicks 104
>   plasticity 97, 120
>   steroids 22, 22*f*, 101, 101*f*
>   training adaptations 17, 18, 20, 21, 21*f*, 82, 94, 94*f*, 95
>   20-minute workout 100, 100*t*
>   weight management 120

hypobaria 45, 165, 165*f*
hypoglycemia 62*t*, 65, 66
hyponatremia 44
hypothermia 164
hypovolemia. *See also* heat
>   altitude exposure 166, 167
>   effects 12, 19, 42-43, 62*t*, 66-67, 67*f*, 133, 147, 156
>   fluid-regulatory mechanisms 41-42, 43, 158*f*
>   guidelines for fluid intake 40, 43, 44, 67
>   hyperthermia 66, 68, 68*f*, 156, 158*f*, 160-161, 162
>   hyponatremia 44

hypoxia 165
hypoxic training 59

I

ibuprofen 102
illness and disease 21, 21*f*, 114, 116, 119, 129. *See also* heat
indirect calorimetry 49, 50, 109-114, 109*f*, 110*f*, 112*t*, 113*f*. *See also* oxygen
individuality 80, 81, 81*f*. *See also* training principles
infancy 172, 172*f*
inflammation 18, 18*f*, 21, 21*f*, 102
injuries
>   anterior cruciate ligament (ACL) injuries 184
>   children 175, 178
>   program design 79, 84, 129, 135

insulin 22, 101
insulin-like growth factor (IGF-1) 22, 101
intensity
>   defining and monitoring 91, 133
>   glycogen depletion and fatigue 64-65, 64f
>   lactate threshold 51, 57, 133, 145, 145*f*

internal respiration 28, 28*f*, 29, 38, 38*f*, 38*t*, 47, 53*f*
interval training 16, 81, 82, 130-133, 131*f*, 149, 150, 176
irisin 111
iron 40*f*, 46*f*, 47, 183
isometric contractions 102, 103*f*

J

jumping 134, 134*f*, 173, 184

K

kettlebell weights 102, 103*f*
kilocalories. *See* Calories
Kipsang Kiprotich, Wilson 144
Krebs cycle 28, 28*f*, 29, 38, 38*f*, 38*t*, 47, 53*f*

L

lactate threshold 51, 57, 145, 145*f*, 180. *See also* anaerobic training

lactic acid 29, 47*f*, 69, 69*f*, 70, 137
lactose 31*f*
leucine 35
liver functions and adaptations 30, 32*f*, 36*f*, 37*f*, 41*f*, 65, 66, 87
Lombardi, Vince 75
low responders 13, 57, 81, 81*f*, 129, 143. *See also* genetics
lungs
>   adaptations to aerobic training 14, 15, 48
>   exchange of oxygen and carbon dioxide 46, 46*f*, 177*f*

M

machine weights 102, 103*f*
macronutrients. *See* carbohydrate; fat; protein; vitamins and minerals
maltodextrin 30
maltose 31*f*
marathon runners 10, 10*f*, 11*t*, 28, 28*f*, 126, 144. *See also* running
mass, muscle. *See* hypertrophy
maturation 172-173, 172*f*, 174, 174*f*
maximal exercise test 50, 133
maximal heart rate 52, 133, 167*f*, 177*f*, 180
maximal oxygen consumption. *See also* aerobic endurance
>   children 176, 177*f*
>   gender differences 57, 143
>   genetics 13, 57, 143
>   lactate threshold connection 51, 57, 145, 145*f*, 180
>   limiting factors 13, 56, 57, 140, 143
>   measures and meaning 49, 50, 139, 140-141
>   older adults 179, 179*f*, 180, 181, 181*f*
>   performance enhancement techniques 58-59
>   testing 51
>   training 49, 50, 50*f*, 51, 54, 55*f*, 56-57, 142, 142*f*

$\dot{V}O_{2peak}$ 53
medulla 55*f*
menopause 173
menstruation 178, 184
metabolic acidosis 62*t*, 69-70, 69*f*. *See also* anaerobic training; lactic acid
metabolic equivalent of training (MET) 49, 50, 112, 112*t*, 133
metabolism. *See* adenosine triphosphate (ATP); Calories
Mexico City 165*f*
Miami (Florida) 165*f*
Mifflin-St. Jeor equation 115*t*
milk 35, 99
minerals and vitamins 29, 39-40, 39*f*, 40*t*
mitochondria 5, 8*f*, 10*f*, 12, 12*f*, 14, 20, 29, 143, 181
mode 91
monosaccharides 30, 31*f*. *See also* carbohydrate
morning workouts 65

motivation 62, 68, 72*f*, 74, 89, 129, 144, 146*f*
motor skills 174, 174*f*
motor units 6, 6*f*, 8-9, 8*f*, 10, 17
mountaineers 45, 59. *See also* altitude
mountain sickness 169, 169*f*
Mt. Everest 45, 165, 165*f*
muscles. *See also* hypertrophy; strength training
>   altitude exposure 167*f*
>   children 173, 175, 177*f*
>   contraction process 6-9, 6*f*, 7*f*, 8*f*
>   cramps 19, 160-161
>   fast-twitch versus slow-twitch fibers 10-11, 10*f*, 11*t*
>   genetics 11, 12*f*, 94, 94*f*
>   hormones 22, 22*f*
>   older adults 179, 179*f*, 180-181, 180*f*, 182
>   oxygen transport 46-48, 46*f*, 47*f*, 48*f*
>   stretching 11
>   types and structure 4-5, 4f

myelination 174, 174*f*
myofibrils 4*f*, 5, 7*f*, 8*f*, 9, 11, 12, 20, 22*f*, 70*f*, 94, 95, 102
myoglobin 47
myosin 4*f*, 5, 7*f*, 8*f*, 9, 11, 12, 20, 22*f*, 70*f*, 94, 95, 102

N

nervous system
>   cardiovascular system function 55*f*
>   development in children 174, 174*f*
>   glucose 30, 66
>   transmission disruption and fatigue 62, 62*t*, 71, 71*f*

nitrates 59
nitrogen 45
nonexercise activity thermogenesis (NEAT) 109*f*, 113, 113*f*, 119
nonsteroidal anti-inflammatory drugs (NSAIDs) 102
norepinephrine 53, 164
nuclei 4, 5, 12, 20, 21, 21*f*, 94, 101
nutrition. *See also* hydration; weight management
>   bone health 105-106, 173
>   cramps 19
>   energy stores 36, 37, 37*f*
>   energy to food 23, 108
>   food to energy 24-25, 24*f*, 27, 27*f*, 30-37, 31*f*, 32*f*, 33*f*, 34*t*, 35*f*, 36*f*, 37*f*, 38, 38*f*, 38*t*
>   hypoglycemia 62*t*, 65, 66
>   macronutrient uses other than energy 26
>   pregnancy 183
>   recovery 34-35, 105, 129
>   sports food and drinks 30, 32, 37, 65, 123
>   strength training nutrition 99, 105-106
>   supplements 35, 37, 106, 114, 129, 137, 177
>   training response 12

vegetables and endurance performance 59
vitamins and minerals 39-40, 39f, 40t
water 41-42, 41f, 43, 44, 45, 99, 129

O

obesity 50, 121, 141, 183. *See also* weight management
older adults 50, 52, 105-106, 179-182, 179f, 180f, 181f
oligosaccharides 30. *See also* carbohydrate
ossification 173, 173f
osteoporosis 173
overload 73, 84, 85, 85f, 86, 87-89, 88f, 91. *See also* program design
overtraining 72-74, 72f, 73f, 75, 84, 85, 85f, 89-90, 91
oxidative production of ATP 28, 28f, 29, 38, 38f, 38t, 47, 53f
oxygen. *See also* altitude; $\dot{V}O_{2max}$
    breathing and oxygen supply 45, 59, 165, 165f
    delivery to muscles 46-48, 46f, 47f, 48f, 56, 140
    metabolic needs 49, 50, 52-53
    oxygen deficit versus excess postexercise oxygen consumption 53, 53f
    performance enhancement techniques 58-59, 147, 168

P

performance capacity 179, 180
perimysium 4f, 5
periodization 80, 84, 88-89, 88f, 91, 135. *See also* training principles
phenolphthalein 114
phosphocreatine (PCr) system 27, 28, 28f, 29, 38, 38f, 38t, 53f, 62t, 63, 63f
photosynthesis 23, 45, 108
physical activity energy expenditure 49, 109f, 112-113, 112t, 113f
pickle juice 19
Pikes Peak 165f
placebo effect 59
planks 103f
plasmalemma 7f, 8, 8f. *See also* satellite cells
plasticity 97, 120
plyometrics 134, 134f, 173, 184
polysaccharides 31. *See also* carbohydrate
power 91, 126, 127f. *See also* speed and power training
precooling aids 69, 157. *See also* hyperthermia
program design. *See also* aerobic endurance; speed and power training; strength training; weight management
    adaptation and overload 73, 84, 85, 85f, 86, 87-89, 88f, 91
    children 172, 175, 176, 177f, 178
    key terms 91-92

older adults 182
participant factors which affect program design 79, 86, 86t
training principles 80-85, 81f, 85f
progressive overload 73, 84, 85, 85f, 86, 87-89, 88f, 91. *See also* program design
protein
    breakdown and uses in the body 26, 27, 27f, 34, 34t, 35f, 36f
    daily intake and recovery guidelines 34-35, 99
    essential and nonessential amino acids 34, 34t
    fat loss and muscle management 120
    functional protein adaptations from training 75, 87-88
    strength training nutrition 99, 105-106
    synthesis 23, 108
Prozac 114
puberty 21, 96, 172f, 173, 174f, 175, 176
pulmonary function. *See* lungs
push-ups 103f

R

radiation 156, 156f, 157f. *See also* heat
rating of perceived exertion (RPE) 133
reaction time 174f
recovery
    nutrition 34-35, 105, 129
    oxygen 59
    training 12, 72-74, 72f, 73f, 84, 85, 85f, 89-90, 91
red blood cells 46f, 47, 47f, 57, 58, 59 147
reflexes 6, 71f, 128, 179f
repetitions 91
resistance training. *See* strength training
respiration
    external respiration 46-48, 46f, 47f, 48f
    internal respiration 28, 28f, 29, 38, 38f, 38t, 47
respiratory exchange ratio (RER) 52-53
rest. *See* recovery; sleep
resting metabolic rate (RMR) 49, 50, 109f, 110, 110f, 114, 115, 115t, 119, 120
reversibility 80, 83, 83f
running. *See also* aerobic endurance
    altitude training 59
    bone health 173, 181
    children 178
    distance runners 10, 10f, 11t, 28, 28f, 126, 144
    energy cost of running 49, 112, 112t
    older adults 181, 181f
    sprint runners 10, 10f, 11t, 28, 28f, 29, 64, 65, 152
    tapering 89

treadmill running 65, 65f, 112-113
type of running and muscle glycogen depletion 65, 65f

S

salt 19, 40, 44, 158f, 161
sarcolemma 7f, 8, 8f. *See also* satellite cells
sarcopenia 179, 179f, 180-181, 180f
sarcoplasmic reticulum 5, 7f, 8-9, 8f, 10f
satellite cells 20, 21, 21f, 134
sea level 45, 59, 165, 165f
sedentary lifestyle 139, 141f, 179f
set point for body weight 119
sets 92
sex. *See* gender differences
shin splints 84
shivering 163, 163f, 164
shot-putters 11t
sibutramine 114
sildenafil 114
sleep 19, 112t, 129
sliding filaments 4f, 5, 7f, 8f, 9, 11, 12, 20, 22f, 70f, 94, 95, 102
slow-twitch muscle fibers
    adaptations to training 14, 16
    characteristics and function 10-11, 10f, 11t
soccer training session 131f
sodium 19, 40, 40f, 44, 158f, 161
sodium bicarbonate 70
sodium citrate 70
softball training session 130
soreness 18, 18f, 21, 21f, 102
specificity 80, 82-83, 130, 131-132. *See also* training principles
speed and power training. *See also* anaerobic training; training principles
    aerobic connection 128, 131, 132
    cross-training considerations 135
    intensity 133
    interval training 130-132, 131f
    neuromuscular adaptations 125, 128
    nutrition guidelines 34-35, 137
    plyometrics 134, 134f, 173, 184
    sample training session 136, 136t
    speed versus power 91, 92, 126, 127f
sport drinks 30, 32, 37, 65, 123
sprint runners. *See also* speed and power training
    endurance capacity 152
    energy systems 28, 28f, 29
    glycogen depletion 64, 65
    muscle composition 10, 10f, 11t
stability balls 102, 103f
starches 31. *See also* carbohydrate
steroids 22, 22f, 101, 101f
strength
    defining 92
    older adults 179, 179f, 180
strength training. *See also* training principles

strength training *(continued)*
　　adaptations 3, 12-13, 12*f*, 14-15, 16, 17, 20, 21, 21*f*, 82, 88, 94*f*, 95
　　beginning gains and plasticity 6, 94, 97
　　children 174*f*, 175
　　circuit training 131
　　cross-training considerations 135, 148, 149, 151
　　delayed-onset muscle soreness (DOMS) 18, 18*f*, 21, 21*f*, 102
　　eccentric training 18, 82, 102, 103*f*, 134, 134*f*
　　energy cost 112*t*
　　equipment and exercises 102, 103*f*
　　females 96, 96*f*, 183
　　general guidelines 75, 98-99, 102
　　gimmicks 104
　　muscle fiber composition of weightlifters 11*t*
　　nutrition 34-35, 99, 105-106
　　older adults 180-181, 180*f*, 182
　　plyometrics 134, 134*f*, 173, 184
　　restricting blood flow 59, 104
　　steroids 22, 22*f*, 101, 101*f*
　　20-minute workout 100, 100*t*
stress
　　hormones 52, 53, 89, 164
　　training load 73, 84, 85, 85*f*, 86, 87-89, 88*f*, 91
stretching and flexibility 11, 13, 135, 146*f*, 148, 162, 180, 182
stroke volume 14, 43, 52, 54, 66, 142*f*, 176, 177*f*, 180
success in sport, determining factors 129
sucrose 31*f*
sugars. *See* carbohydrate
supplements 35, 37, 106, 114, 129, 137, 177
sweating
　　children and older adults 177*f*, 181
　　environmental factors 158*f*, 163
　　fluid needs and hyponatremia 41, 43, 44
　　hot yoga 162
　　mineral loss 19, 40, 161
　　temperature regulation 156, 157*f*, 158*f*, 159-160, 159*f*
　　weight loss 42-43, 67, 67*f*
swimmers
　　characteristics 11*t*, 164
　　training 19, 59, 82, 89, 112, 112*t*, 178
synaptic cleft 7*f*, 8
systolic pressure 56. *See also* blood pressure

T
tapering 89, 92, 149
taurine 37

temperature. *See* cold; heat
tennis 112, 112*t*
testosterone
　　effects 22, 22*f*, 184
　　gender differences 13, 96, 184
　　steroids 22, 22*f*, 101, 101*f*
thermic effect of food (TEF) 109, 109*f*, 110, 119
thermodynamics 108
thermogenesis 109
titin 9, 11
training principles. *See also* program design
　　individuality 80, 81, 81*f*
　　overload 73, 84, 85, 85*f*, 86, 87-89, 88*f*, 91
　　reversibility 80, 83, 83*f*
　　specificity 80, 82-83, 130, 131-132
　　variation principle 80, 84, 88-89, 88*f*, 91, 135
training variables 92
training volume 92
transverse tubules (T-tubules) 7*f*, 8, 8*f*
treadmill running 65, 65*f*, 112-113
triamterine 114
triathletes 11*t*
tricarboxylic acid 28, 28*f*, 29, 38, 38*f*, 38*t*, 47, 53*f*
triglycerides. *See* fat
troponin and tropomyosin 7*f*, 70*f*, 94
type II muscle fibers
　　adaptations to training 16
　　characteristics and function 10-11, 10*f*, 11*t*
　　older adults 179*f*, 181
type I muscle fibers
　　adaptations to training 14, 16
　　characteristics and function 10-11, 10*f*, 11*t*

U
U.S. Centers for Disease Control and Prevention (CDC) 182
U.S. Food and Drug Administration 114

V
Valsalva maneuvers 183
variation principle 80, 84, 88-89, 88*f*, 91, 102, 103*f*, 135. *See also* training principles
ventilatory threshold 51, 57, 145, 145*f*, 180. *See also* anaerobic training; lactic acid
ventilatory volume 177*f*
Viagra 114
vibration platforms 102
vitamins and minerals 29, 39-40, 39*f*, 40*t*
$\dot{V}O_{2max}$. *See also* aerobic endurance
　　children 176, 177*f*
　　gender differences 57, 143

genetics 13, 57, 143
lactate threshold connection 51, 57, 145, 145*f*, 180
limiting factors 13, 56, 57, 140, 143
measures and meaning 49, 50, 139, 140-141
older adults 179, 179*f*, 180, 181, 181*f*
performance enhancement techniques 58-59
testing 51
training 49, 50, 50*f*, 51, 54, 55*f*, 56-57, 142, 142*f*
$\dot{V}O_{2peak}$ 53

W
walking 112*t*
warm-ups 157
water
　　cold-water exposure 164
　　hydration 41-42, 41*f*, 43, 44, 45, 99, 129
weightlifting. *See* strength training
weight management. *See also* nutrition; training principles
　　Calorie expenditure 49, 50, 109-114, 109*f*, 110*f*, 112*t*, 113*f*, 115, 115*t*, 119, 120
　　Calorie input 108, 108*f*, 109, 183
　　children 176
　　disordered eating 114, 116, 119
　　energy balance versus energy availability 107-109, 108*f*, 109*f*, 116-117, 117*t*, 179
　　energy efficiency versus energy deficiency 109*f*, 110-111, 116, 117*t*, 184
　　estimating daily energy needs 50, 114, 115, 115*t*
　　exercising while eating versus fasting 123-124, 123*f*, 124*f*
　　factors influencing weight loss 118-119, 118*f*
　　fat-burning zone 122, 122*f*
　　fat types 110-111, 121
　　high-fat and low-carbohydrate diets 124, 124*f*
　　losing fat and keeping muscle 120-121
　　older adults 179, 179*f*
　　severe Calorie restriction 114, 116, 119, 120
　　speed and power training 126
　　supplements 114
wind 156, 157, 157*f*, 163*f*
work 92
workload 92

Y
yoga 162, 182

Bob Murray, PhD, FACSM, is the cofounder of the Gatorade Sports Science Institute (GSSI) and served as its director from 1985 to 2008. Murray oversaw a broad program of GSSI- and university-based research in exercise science and sport nutrition that set industry standards and consumer expectations for science-based product efficacy. Murray has been an invited speaker at professional meetings worldwide.

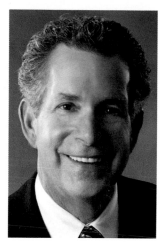

A native of Pittsburgh, Murray earned his BS and MEd degrees in physical education at Slippery Rock University. He was an assistant professor of physical education and head swimming coach at Oswego State University from 1974 to 1977 before earning his PhD in exercise physiology from Ohio State University. He then was assistant and associate professor of physical education at Boise State University from 1980 to 1985 before relocating to Chicago to cofound the Gatorade Sports Science Institute. An author of numerous publications in scientific texts and journals, Murray is a fellow of the American College of Sports Medicine and an honorary member of the Academy of Nutrition and Dietetics.

W. Larry Kenney, PhD, is the Marie Underhill Noll Chair in Human Performance and a professor of physiology and kinesiology at Pennsylvania State University at University Park. He received his PhD in physiology from Penn State in 1983. Working at Noll Laboratory, Kenney is researching the effects of aging and disease states such as hypertension on the control of blood flow to human skin and has been continuously funded by NIH since 1983. He also studies the effects of heat, cold, and dehydration on various aspects of health, exercise, and athletic performance as well as the biophysics of heat exchange between humans and the environment. He is the author of more than 200 papers, books, book chapters, and other publications.

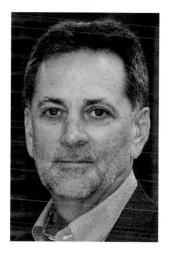

Kenney was president of the American College of Sports Medicine from 2003 to 2004. He is a fellow of the American College of Sports Medicine and is active in the American Physiological Society.

For his service to the university and his field, Kenney was awarded Penn State's Faculty Scholar Medal, the Evan G. and Helen G. Pattishall Distinguished Research Career Award, and the Pauline Schmitt Russell Distinguished Research Career Award. He was awarded the American College of Sports Medicine's New Investigator Award in 1987 and the Citation Award in 2008.

Kenney has been a member of the editorial and advisory boards for several journals, including *Medicine and Science in Sports and Exercise*, *Current Sports Medicine Reports* (inaugural board member), *Exercise and Sport Sciences Reviews*, *Journal of Applied Physiology*, *Human Performance*, *Fitness Management*, and *ACSM's Health & Fitness Journal* (inaugural board member). He is also an active grant reviewer for the National Institutes of Health and many other organizations. He and his wife, Patti, have three children, all of whom are or were Division I college athletes.

3702002